Indian
head massage
A beginner's guide

Indian head massage

A beginner's guide

Denise Whichello Brown

Published by SILVERDALE BOOKS
An imprint of Bookmart Ltd
Registered number 2372865
Trading as Bookmart Ltd
Desford Road
Enderby
Leicester LE19 4AD

D&S Books Ltd
Kerswell,
Parkham Ash, Bideford
Devon, England
EX39 5PR

e-mail us at:-
enquiries@dsbooks.fsnet.co.uk

This edition printed 2002

ISBN 1-85605-680-5

Creative Director: Sarah King
Editor: Clare Haworth-Maden
Project editor: Yvonne Worth
Photographer: Colin Bowling
Designer: David Jones

Printed in China

1 3 5 7 9 10 8 6 4 2

Contents

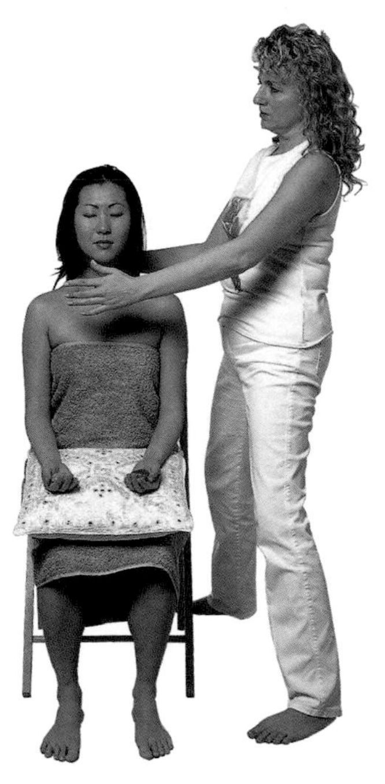

The Origins of Indian Head Massage

INDIAN HEAD MASSAGE is an ancient art. Its origins lie in the traditional Indian system of medicine known as Ayurveda, the most ancient form of healing, whose texts, which date back thousands of years, detail the importance of massage. A Sanskrit word, Ayurveda is derived from two roots: *ayur*, which means 'life', and *veda*, which means 'knowledge'. Ayurveda is thus the science of life that stresses the importance of the holistic principle in balancing the body, mind and spirit and the promotion of health and longevity by using the inherent principles of nature to bring the body back into equilibrium. The Ayurvedic approach to life is therefore recognising your true nature and living according to your true self.

The five elements and the three *doshas*

ACCORDING TO AYURVEDA, the structural aspect of the body is made up of the five elements: earth, air, fire, water and ether.

The functional aspect of the body is governed by the three *doshas*, namely *vata*, *pitta* and *kapha*, which are present in every cell, tissue and organ of the body. Every person's body is made up of a unique combination of these three *doshas*, which can change in accordance with one's diet, lifestyle, climate, emotions and other factors. According to Ayurveda, disease is caused by an imbalance of the *vata*, *pitta* and *kapha doshas*, an imbalance that may be caused by a variety of internal and external factors. The Ayurvedic practitioner will therefore recommend specific lifestyle and nutritional changes to help the individual to reduce the *dosha* that has become excessive. Herbs, cleansing, meditation, yoga and massage with therapeutic oils are also prescribed to achieve a balanced body and thus maintain health.

The qualities bestowed by *vata*, *pitta* and *kapha* are as follows.

Vata qualities

Vata is a combination of the air and ether elements. *Vata* is dry, light, cold, active, mobile, subtle and astringent.

AIR

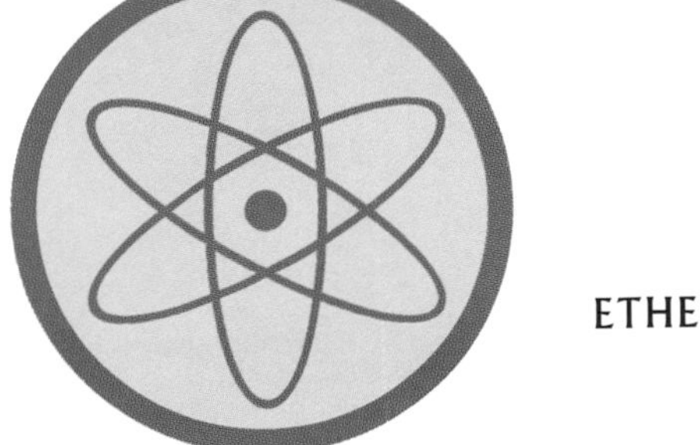

ETHER

- If a person has excessive *vata* in his or her constitution, its dry quality will result in a tendency to have dry hair and skin, as well as a dry colon and consequently constipation.
- As a result of its light quality, a *vata* person will have a light body frame and will therefore be thin.

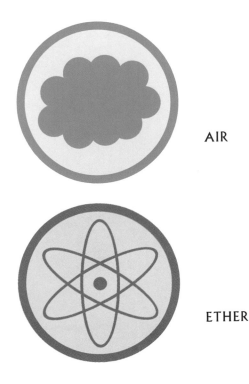

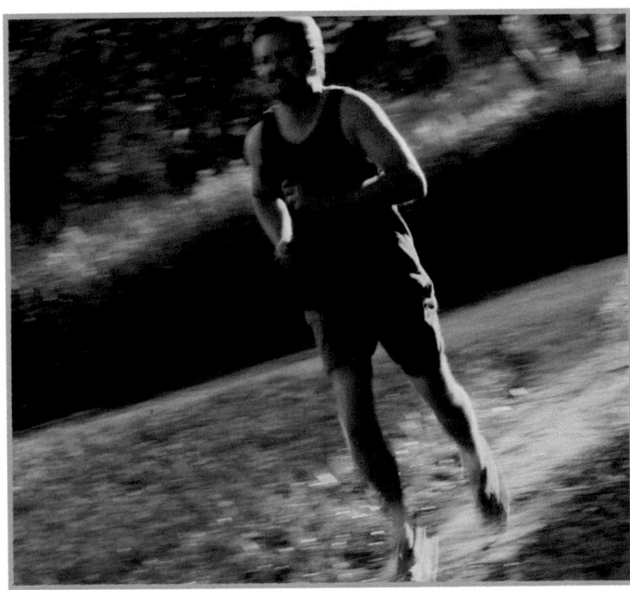

A *vata* person finds it difficult to sit still and will love physical exercise such as jogging.

- On account of *vata's* cold quality, a *vata* person will have cold hands and feet and poor circulation, causing him or her to prefer the warmth of the summer to the coldness of the winter.
- Because of *vata's* active, mobile qualities, *vata* people love exercise, such as jogging, and do not like sitting still.
- *Vata's* subtle quality creates feelings of fear and nervousness, while its clear quality can result in clairvoyance.
- Because *vata* is astringent, a *vata* individual may experience a dry, almost choking, sensation in his or her throat.

In character, *vata* people are very active, finding it difficult to sit still. They may have a tendency to be anxious and fearful.

In general, *vata* people tend to suffer from nervous, muscular and rheumatic disorders, insomnia, dry skin, constipation, poor circulation, tension headaches and feelings of anxiety and worry.

Pitta qualities

Pitta is a combination of the fire and water elements. It is hot, sharp, light, liquid, sour and oily.

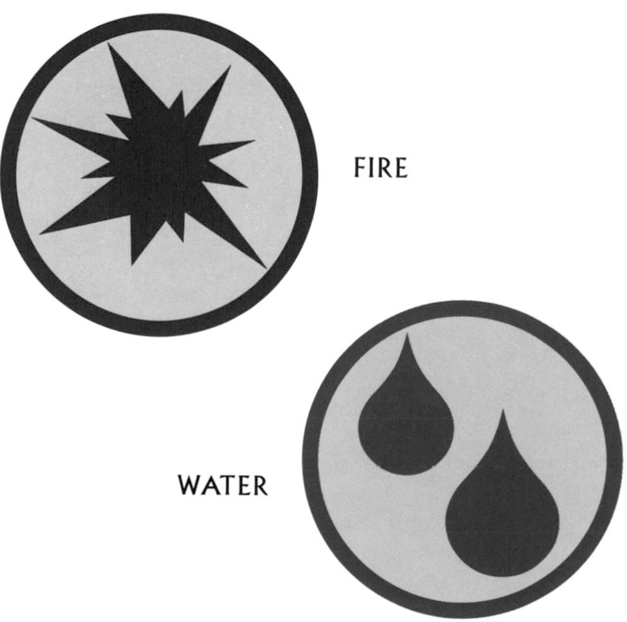

- Due to its hot quality, a *pitta* individual has a slightly warmer body temperature than a *vata* person, and will also perspire more easily, producing a strong smell. A *pitta* person also has a powerful appetite, causing him or her to become irritable when hungry, and cannot easily skip meals.
- *Pitta's* sharp quality gives rise to sharp physical features, such as a pointed nose and teeth, as well as sharp mental qualities, such as a keen intellect and good memory.
- As a result of its light quality, *pitta* individuals have moderately sized body frames and do not like bright light.
- Due to *pitta's* oily quality, *pitta* types have soft, oily skin, straight hair and liquid faeces. They have a tendency to mature early, so that their hair may turn prematurely grey or they may even lose their hair at a relatively young age.

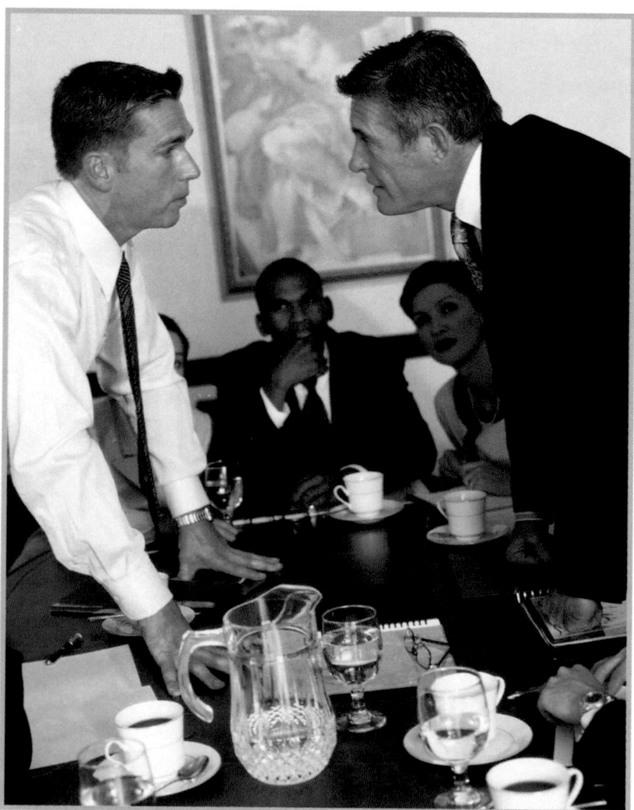

Pitta people have a tendency to control and dominate.

In character, *pitta* people are leaders and organisers. They are ambitious and competitive perfectionists who, due to their controlling personalities, may try to dominate and criticise others.

In general, *pitta* people have a tendency to develop inflammatory diseases, coronary disease, stomach ulcers, psoriasis and herpes.

Kapha qualities

Kapha is a combination of earth and water. Its qualities are heavy, slow and static, cool, oily and liquid, thick, dense and cloudy.

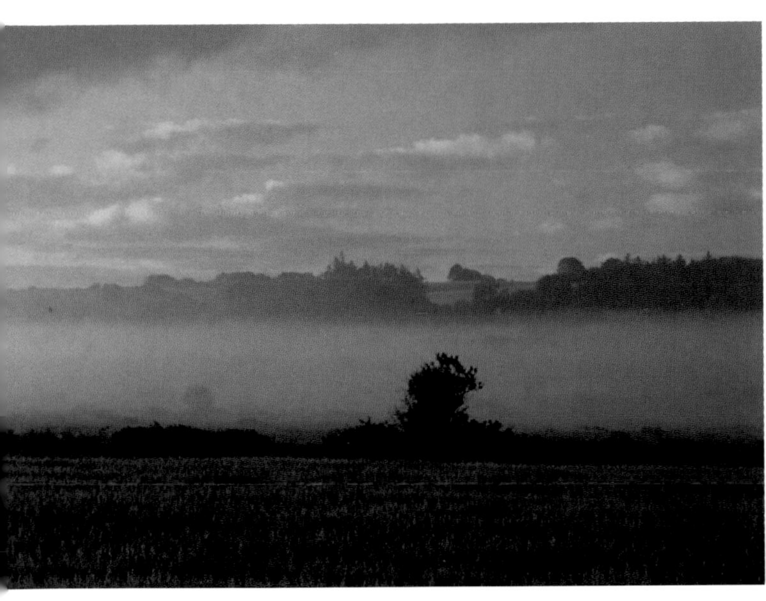

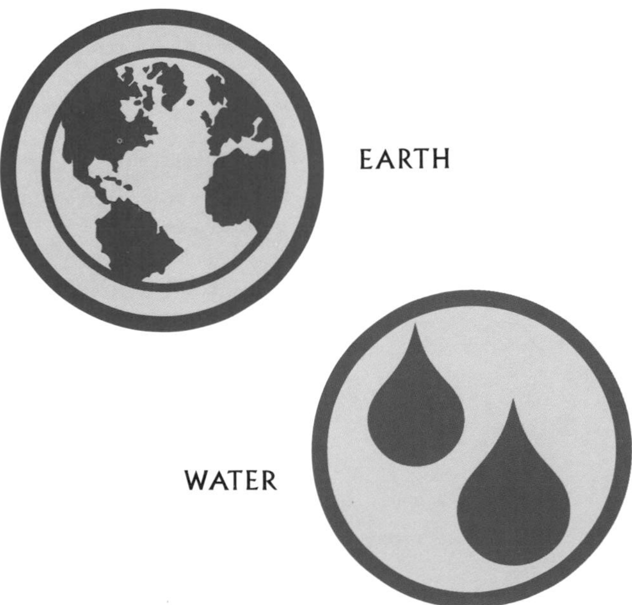

- As a result of *kapha's* heavy quality, *kapha* individuals have heavy bones and muscles and a tendency to put on weight easily.
- Due to *kapha's* slow quality, a *kapha* person has a slow metabolism and digestion. These individuals love to eat especially sweet things. In addition, this quality of slowness causes *kapha* individuals to move, as well as eat, slowly. They are not very enthusiastic about exercising – in fact, under *kapha's* static influence, they prefer to do nothing at all.
- *Kapha's* cool, oily and liquid qualities result in *kapha* individuals having cold and clammy skin, while its characteristics of thickness and density bestow thick, wavy hair.
- Due to *kapha's* cloudy quality, *kapha* people are slow to rise in the morning and, because they feel lethargic and sleepy, they usually need caffeine to get them going.

In character, *kapha* people are very loving and compassionate.

In general, *kapha* individuals tend to suffer from excess weight, lethargy, congestion, coughs, sinus problems and colds.

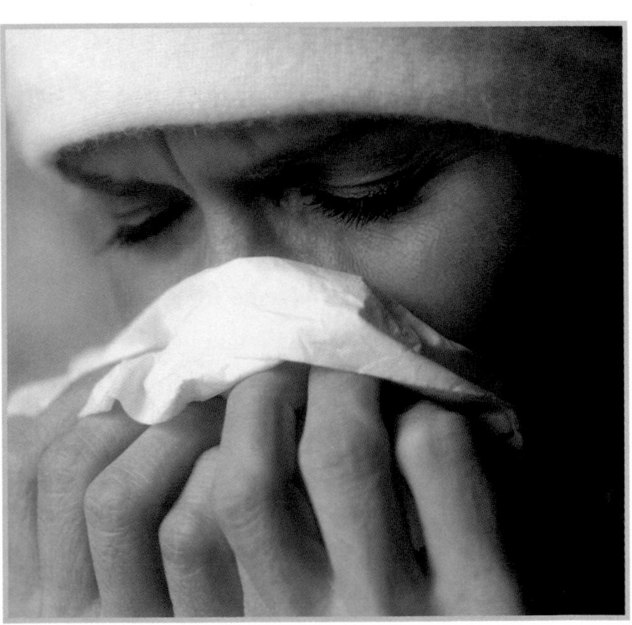

The importance of massage in India

MASSAGE PLAYS A CENTRAL ROLE in Indian family life. An integral part of the everyday routine, it is highly recommended for both men and women in order to balance the *doshas* and thus promote optimum health. Expectant mothers are massaged throughout their pregnancy and for a minimum of forty days after the birth of their baby, while babies are massaged every day from birth to encourage the bonding process. When children are three years old, they are massaged once or twice a week until they are six, and from the age of seven they are encouraged to learn the massage techniques to enable them to perform treatments on members of their family. In India, almost everyone both gives and receives massage. It is traditional, for example, for a bride and groom to receive a massage prior to their wedding ceremony, not only to relax them, but because it is thought to promote health, stamina, beauty and even fertility.

Indian head massage was originally developed by women as part of their grooming routine to keep their hair strong and in beautiful condition and their scalp healthy (and, indeed, the long, lustrous and glossy hair of Indian women is much admired). For men, a visit to the barber will always include a head massage, otherwise known as a champissage, barbers having developed an invigorating massage designed to stimulate their clients' scalps. (Interestingly, the Western word 'shampoo' is derived from the Hindi word *champi*, which means 'having your head massaged'.)

Indian head massage skills are passed on from generation to generation: daughters learn it from their mothers and sons from their families or barber fathers. Indian head massages follow a fixed routine, and each family will have its own distinct techniques to suit different members of the family and for particular occasions. Not only are head massages performed at home and at the barber's shop, they are readily available on the beaches, in the markets and on street corners.

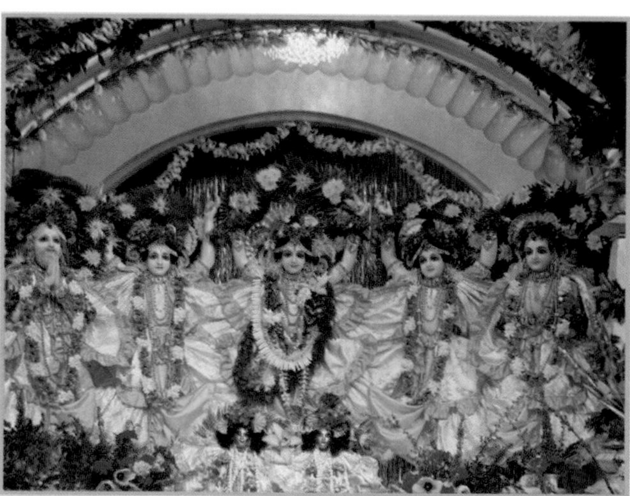

Massage is an important part of traditional Indian life.

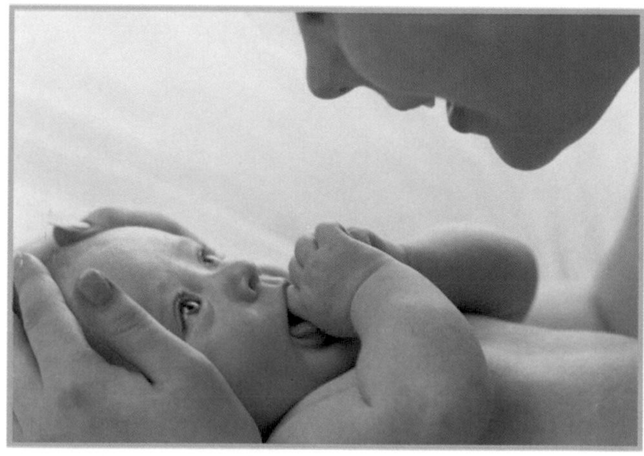

Babies can be massaged every day from birth.

Although Indian head massage was introduced to the West only recently, it has become one of the most popular holistic therapies. Widely taught in many colleges around the world, it has evolved to include techniques for the upper back, shoulders, upper arms and neck, areas that are very susceptible to stress and tension.

When one considers its advantages, one can see why Indian head massage is such a popular therapy.

It can be carried out anywhere – Indian head massage can be practised in a variety of settings: for instance, at home, in a beauty or hair salon, in a nursing or residential-care home, at an airport or at the workplace.

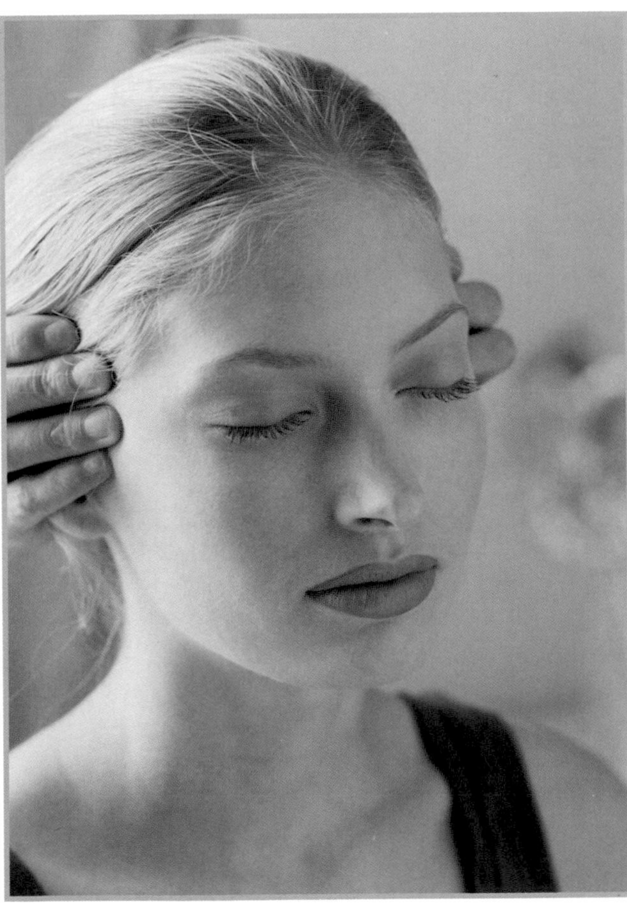

There's no need for the recipient to disrobe – Indian head massage can be performed on a fully clothed client. Not only does this save time at the workplace, it also enables people to enjoy the benefits of massage who would otherwise feel somewhat nervous or embarrassed about taking their clothes off.

No expensive equipment is required – All that you need in order to give an Indian head massage treatment is a chair and a pair of hands. You could use oils (see Chapter 2), but these are entirely optional.

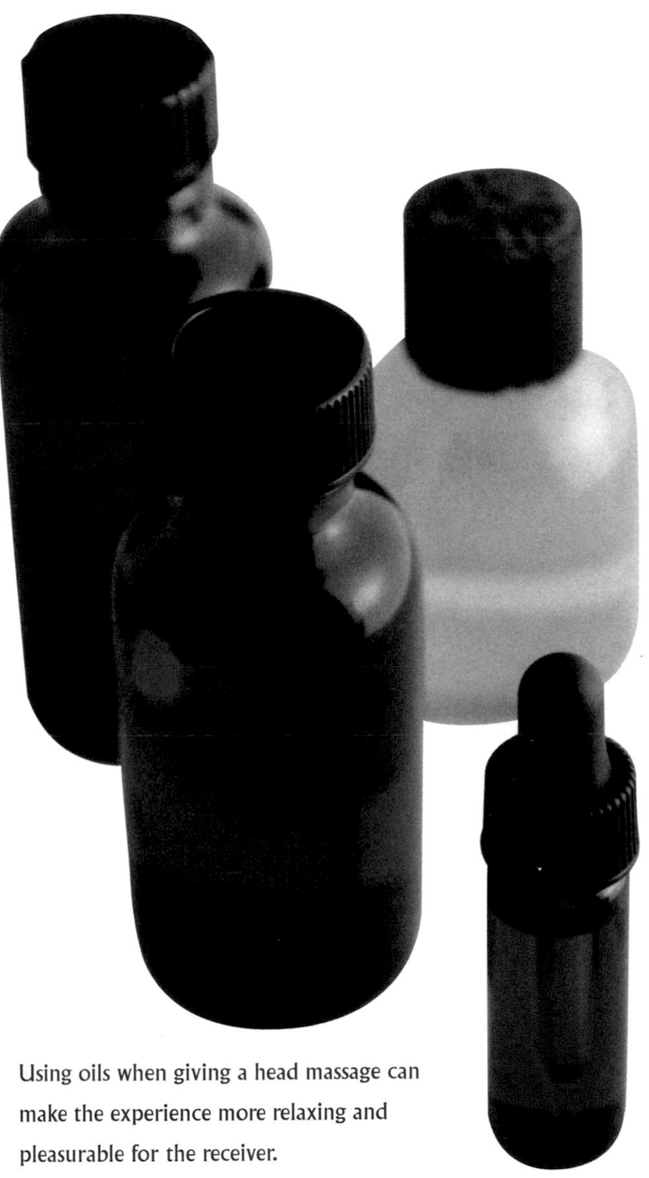

Using oils when giving a head massage can make the experience more relaxing and pleasurable for the receiver.

The treatment is relatively quick to perform – a complete Indian head, neck and shoulder massage may take thirty minutes, yet it is amazing what can be achieved within just a few minutes.

Indian head massage is suitable for all – it is just as suitable for soothing and calming young babies as it is for treating older people.

The benefits of Indian head massage

INDIAN HEAD MASSAGE IS A TRULY HOLISTIC THERAPY that aims to balance the mind, body and spirit, because Indian head massage has a far-reaching effect on every system of the body, it has numerous short- and long-term therapeutic benefits. Although it is impossible to compose an exhaustive list, there follow a few of its countless benefits.

The physical benefits of Indian head massage

The physical benefits of Indian head massage include the following.

THE IMPROVED FUNCTIONING OF THE CIRCULATORY SYSTEM

Fresh blood, carrying oxygen and nutrients, is brought to the tissues, thereby encouraging healing. Indian head massage is also effective when trying to regulate the heartbeat and to reduce high blood pressure.

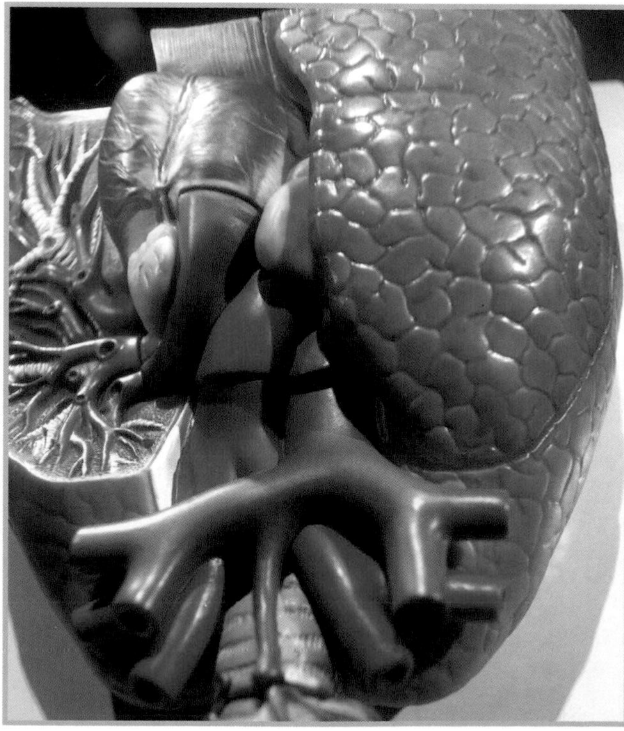

Head massage can help regulate the heartbeat.

THE STIMULATION OF THE LYMPHATIC SYSTEM

Any waste products and toxins that have accumulated in the lymphatic system can be eliminated through Indian head massage. The immune system is also boosted, enabling the body to fight off infection and to recover from illness more rapidly.

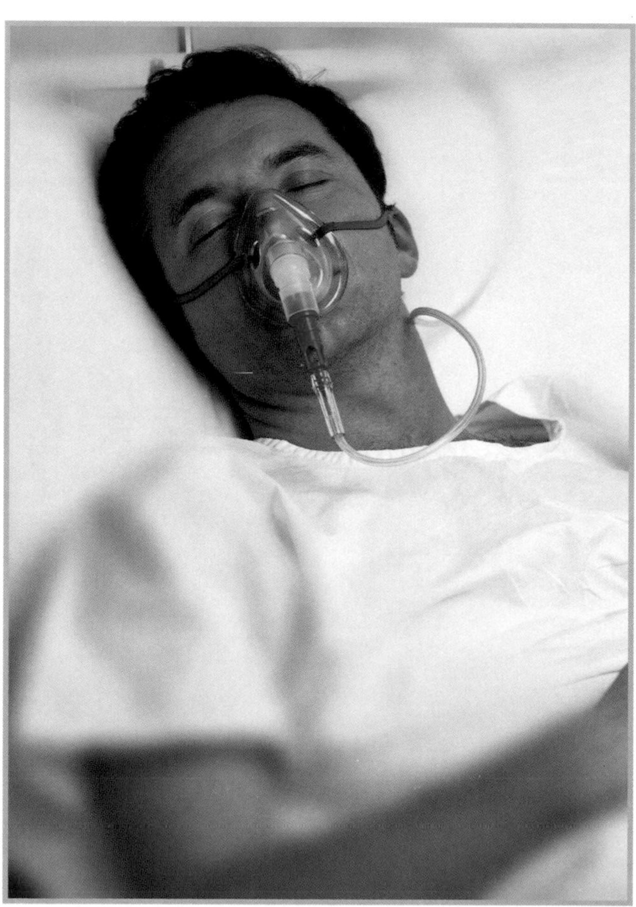

Indian head massage can also promote rapid recovery from illness.

THE RELAXATION OF THE MUSCULAR SYSTEM

Muscular tension in the head, neck, upper back and shoulders is relieved through Indian head massage. Pain and discomfort can be greatly reduced as nodules and adhesions in the muscles are broken down and toxic products eliminated.

INCREASED MOBILITY OF THE JOINTS

Indian head massage is excellent for decreasing stiffness and increasing flexibility in the neck and shoulder area.

RELIEF FROM TENSION HEADACHES AND EYE STRAIN

By massaging the scalp, neck and facial areas, the incidence of tension headaches suffered by the client can be reduced or even eliminated. Tense eye muscles can be relaxed, and eye strain soothed, through Indian head massage.

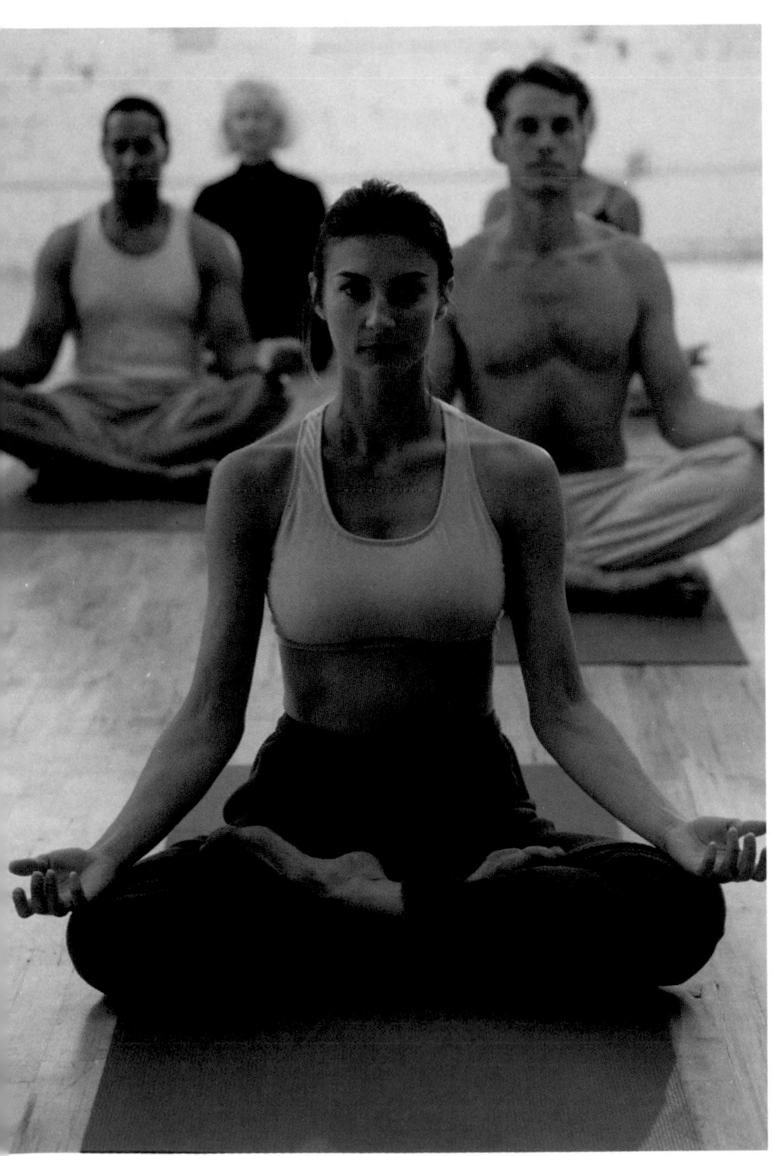

Regular head massage increases flexibility of the joints, and relieves muscle tension.

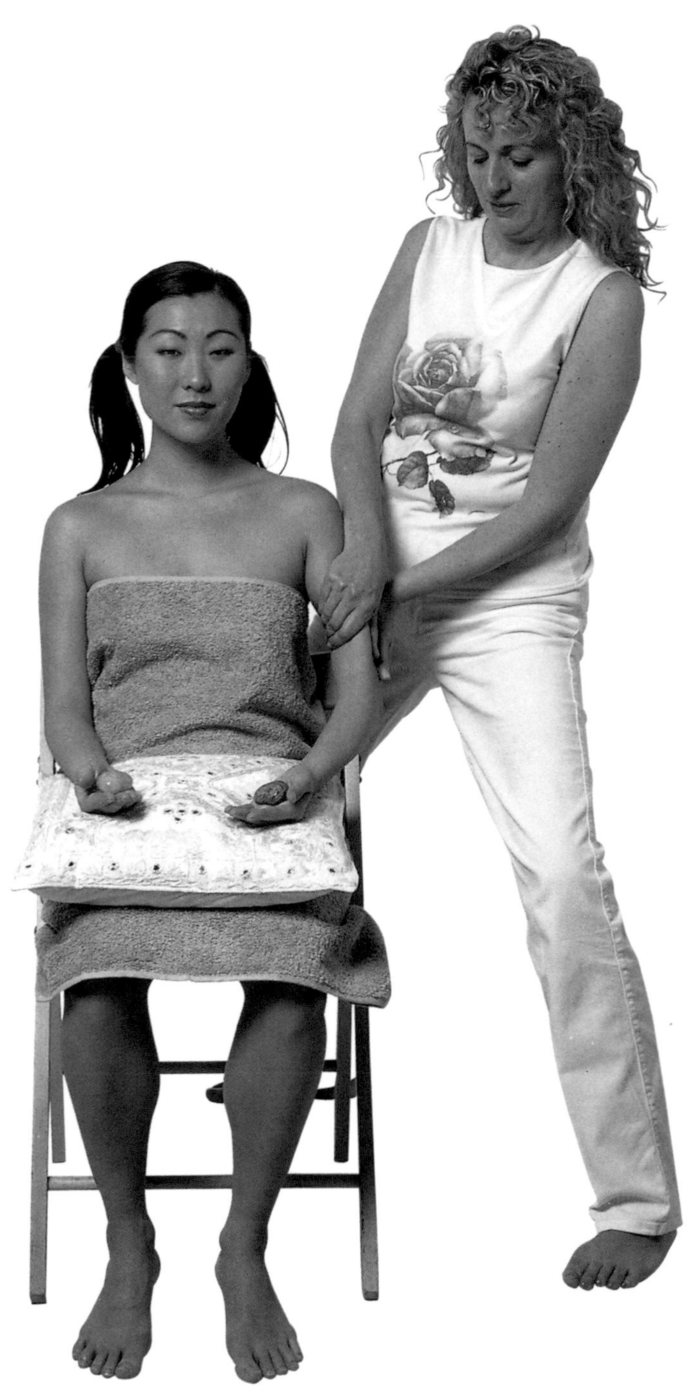

THE PROMOTION OF HAIR GROWTH

The increased flow of blood to the scalp caused by Indian head massage encourages hair growth and improves the condition of the hair.

HEALTHIER-LOOKING SKIN

Because the sweat and sebaceous glands are stimulated by Indian head massage, waste products are more readily eliminated. And because dead skin cells are removed, the condition, colour, texture and tone of the skin improves enormously. The effect can be so dramatically rejuvenating that it takes years off you.

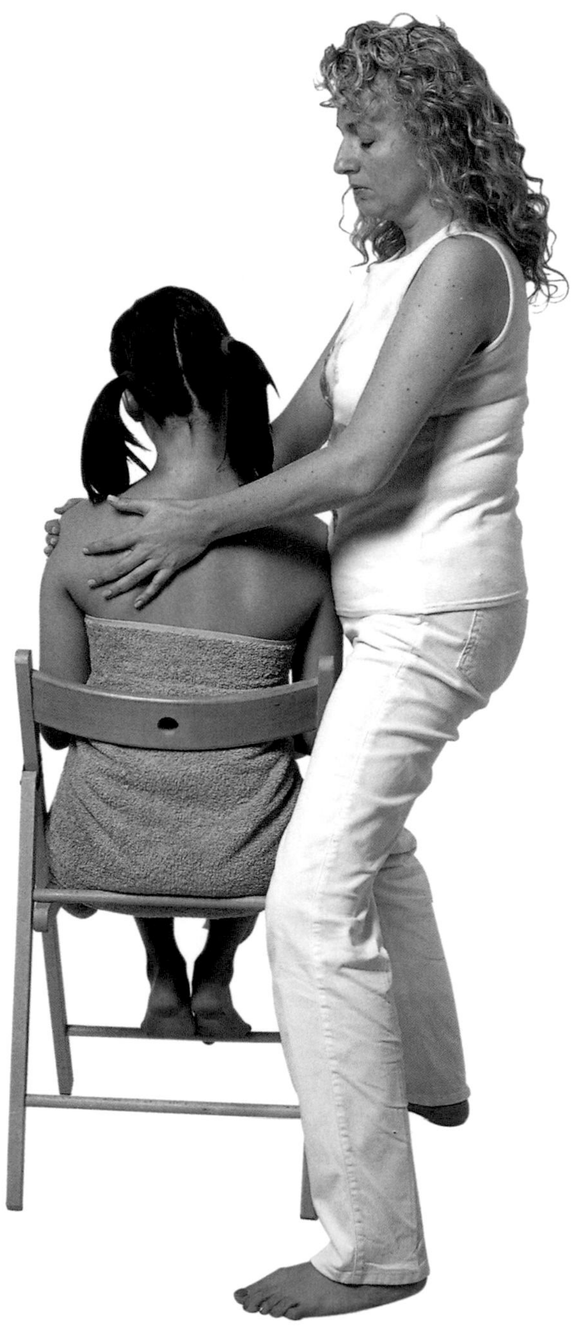

The psychological benefits of Indian head massage

The psychological benefits of Indian head massage include the following.

RELIEF FROM STRESS AND TENSION

Indian head massage is invaluable for de-stressing the whole body, enabling us to cope much more easily with the strains and challenges of everyday life.

A DEEP STATE OF RELAXATION AND RAISED ENERGY LEVELS

A sense of peace and tranquillity is induced during the Indian head massage treatment, followed by a rise in energy levels.

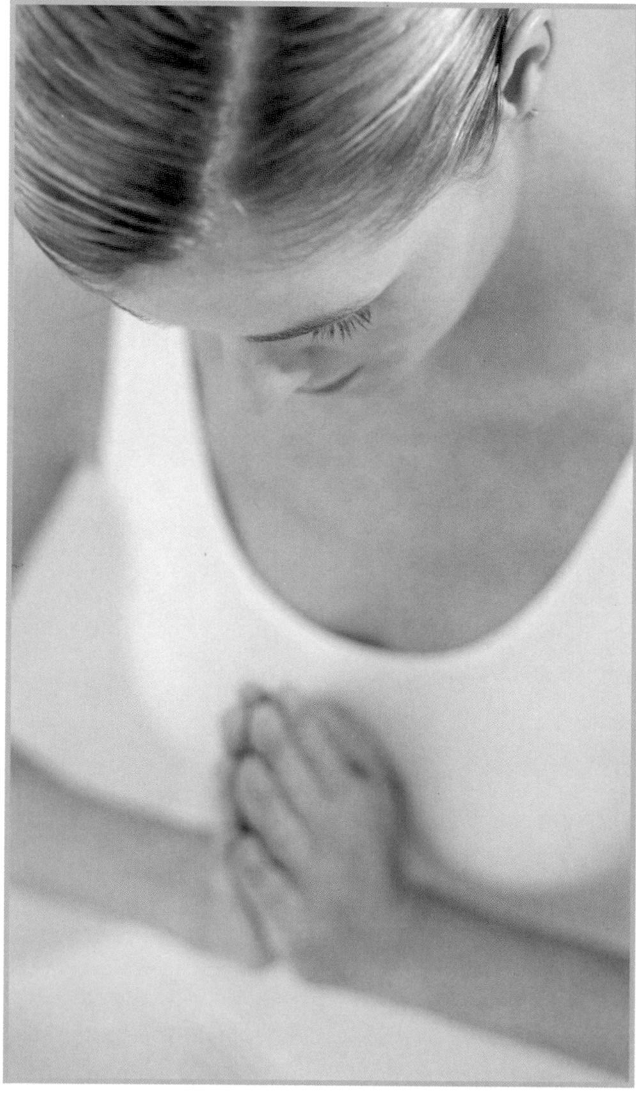

Indian head massage induces peace and tranquillity.

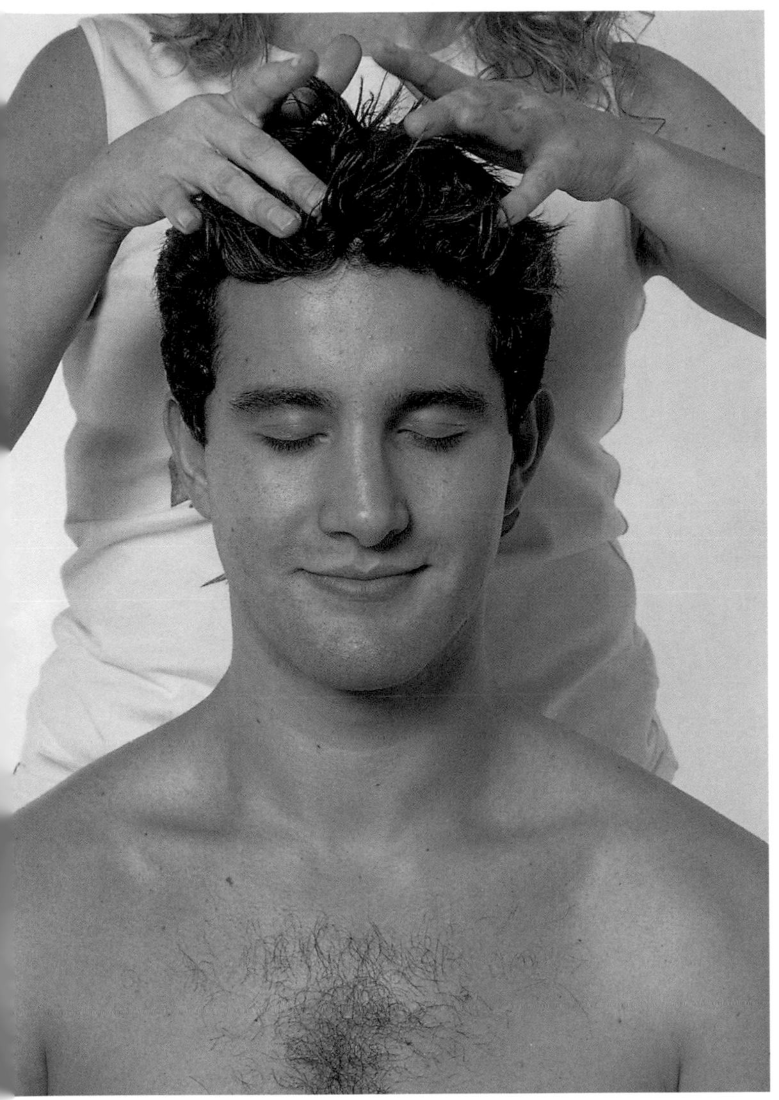

The subtle, spiritual benefits of Indian head massage

The subtle, spiritual benefits of Indian head massage include the following.

THE RELEASE OF BLOCKAGES

Any blockages in the flow of energy known as *Ch'i*, or *prana*, result in health problems. During the Indian head massage treatment, any such blockages are released, enabling energy to flow freely and healing to take place.

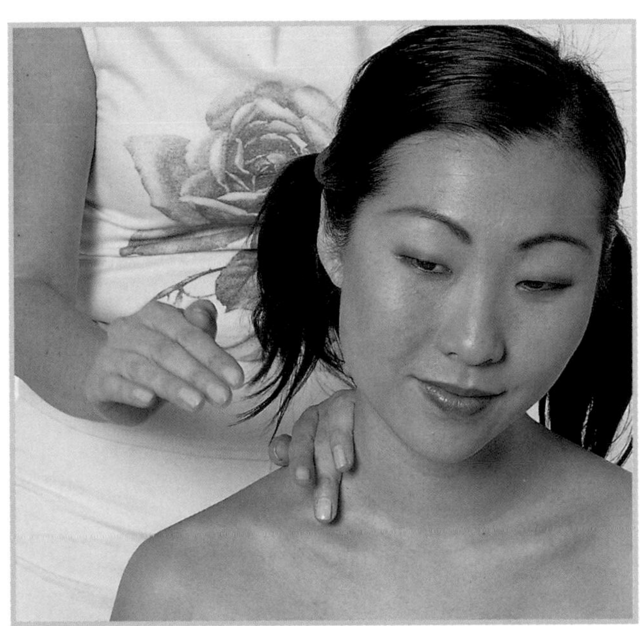

IMPROVED CONCENTRATION

Through Indian head massage, the mind feels alert as mental fatigue is dispelled due to the increased supply of oxygen to the brain. Clarity of thought is thus promoted and creativity increased.

THE LIFTING OF DEPRESSION AND RAISING OF SELF-ESTEEM

Feelings of hopelessness, despair and lack of self-worth are alleviated through Indian head massage, causing recipients to feel uplifted and full of confidence.

THE DISPELLING OF INSOMNIA

Because the mind is calmed and soothed through Indian head massage, an excellent, disturbance-free sleeping pattern is established.

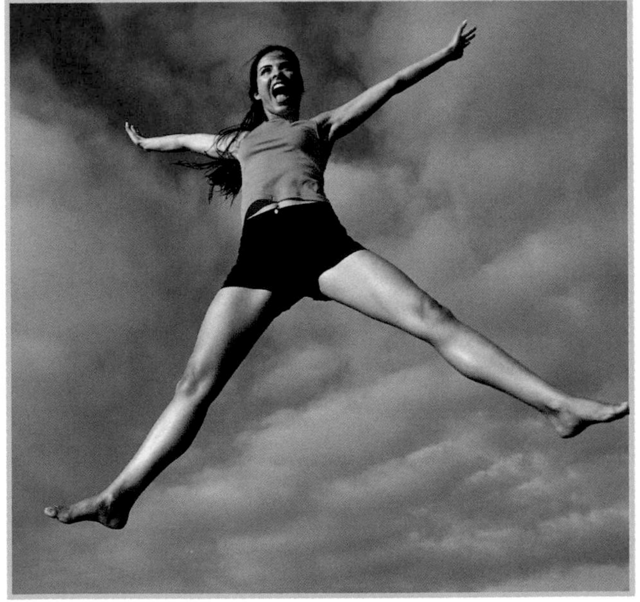

Indian head massage helps release energy, and lift the spirits.

THE BALANCING OF THE CHAKRAS

There are seven major chakras (see Chapter 4), which, when blocked, can cause physical, emotional, mental or spiritual imbalances. At the end of an Indian head massage, the chakras will have been balanced and aligned. (Crystals may also be used to assist the balancing of the chakras.)

ADDITIONAL BENEFITS

In addition to the benefits outlined above, Indian head massage works extremely well alongside orthodox medicine. A gentle and natural treatment, it does not have any adverse side effects.

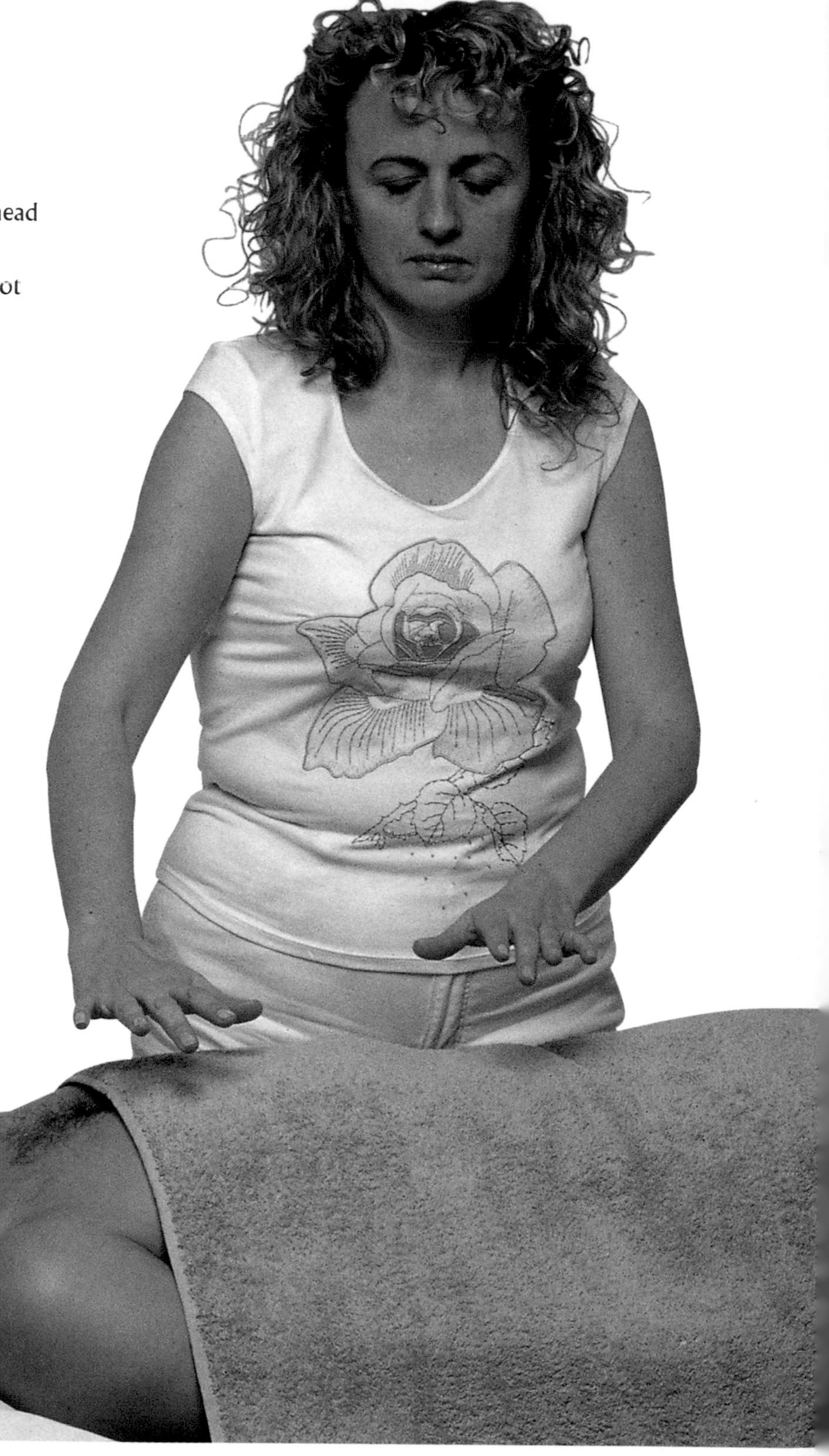

Preparing to give an Indian Head Massage

BEFORE GIVING AN Indian head massage treatment, it is important to create the right ambience. A warm, relaxing and soothing environment will help to ensure the success of your massage.

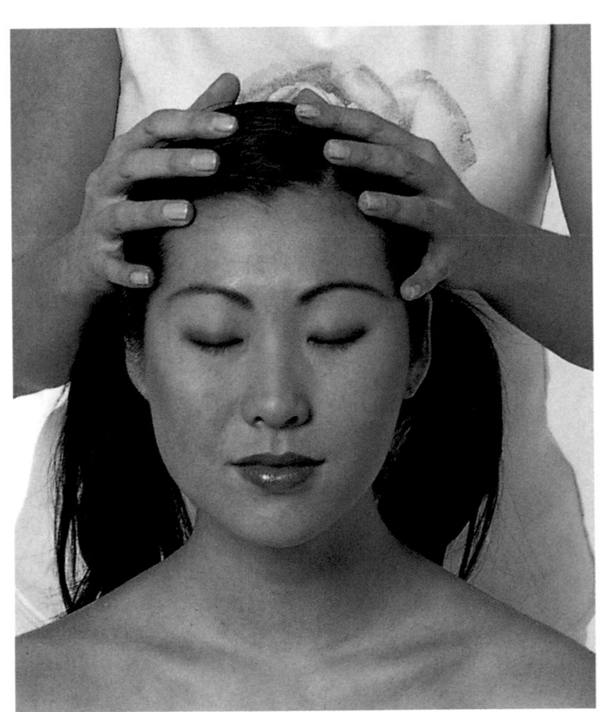

Creating a healing environment

CHOOSE A TIME when you are unlikely to be interrupted. If you are worried about being disturbed, you will be unable to relax and will transfer any feelings of tension to your massage partner. Ensure that any children or pets have been settled down and can safely be left for at least half an hour and perhaps hang a 'Do not disturb!' sign on the door. In addition, turn on the answerphone or unplug the phone.

Temperature

The room should be pleasantly warm, but not stuffy, to encourage your partner to relax. (If you open a window, make sure that there are no draughts.)

Although it is not essential for your partner to remove any clothes, his or her body temperature will drop as the treatment progresses, so have some towels at hand to cover your partner with because the treatment may be spoilt if his or her muscles tighten up in response to feeling cold.

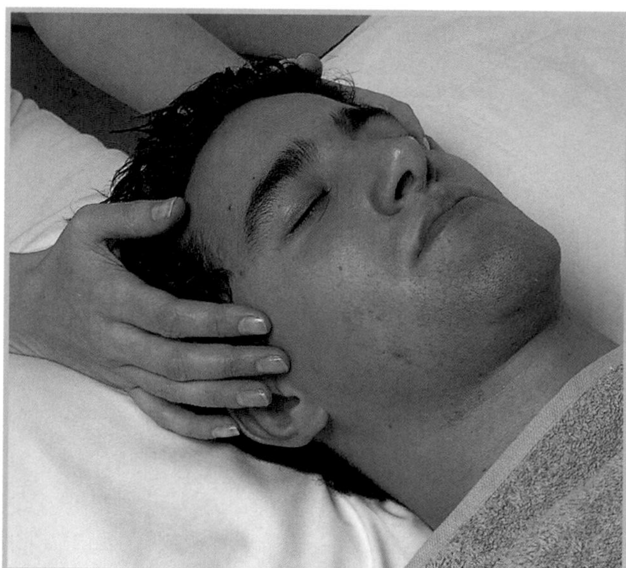

Always cover your partner with towels, as their body temperature will drop during the treatment.

Subtle lighting

Lighting is also an important factor in the success of your treatment. Avoid using bright lights, especially harsh overhead lighting, and instead make use of any dimmer switches, sidelights or, even better, candles. A water feature with candles incorporated into it will transform the mood of the room.

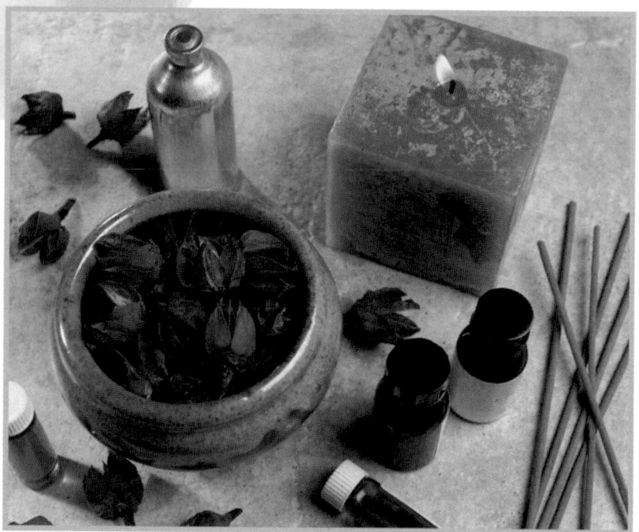

Candles or oil burners help to create the right ambience.

For a special touch, use an oil burner (see also Chapter 2). Simply place a few teaspoons of water into the bowl on top of the oil burner and then add a few drops of essential oil. On lighting the night light underneath, the subtle aroma of the essential oil will start to diffuse into the atmosphere.

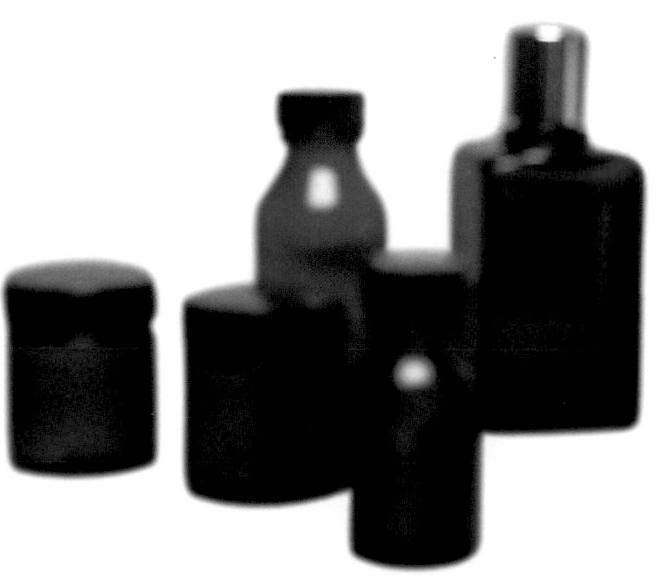

Suitable oils include:

- BERGAMOT – uplifting, antidepressant and balancing;
- CEDARWOOD – calming, soothing, healing and warming;
- CHAMOMILE – deeply relaxing and particularly suitable for treating children;
- CLARY SAGE – intoxicating, sensual and induces feelings of euphoria;
- FRANKINCENSE – mysterious, elevating, rejuvenating and encourages deep breathing;
- GERANIUM – healing, uplifting and harmonising;
- JUNIPER – cleansing, detoxifying and purifying;
- LEMON – antiseptic, cleansing, refreshing and revitalising;
- ROSEMARY – decongestive, restorative and stimulating;
- SANDALWOOD – soothing, sedative, healing and has aphrodisiac qualities.

Soothing music

Music can also impart a feeling of serenity and peace. A wide variety of cassettes and compact discs are available today that have been specially composed for massage and relaxation. Some feature natural sounds, such as running water, rushing winds and the sea.

Check whether your partner has any preferences, and remember that some people may prefer silence, particularly after spending a noisy day at work or with children.

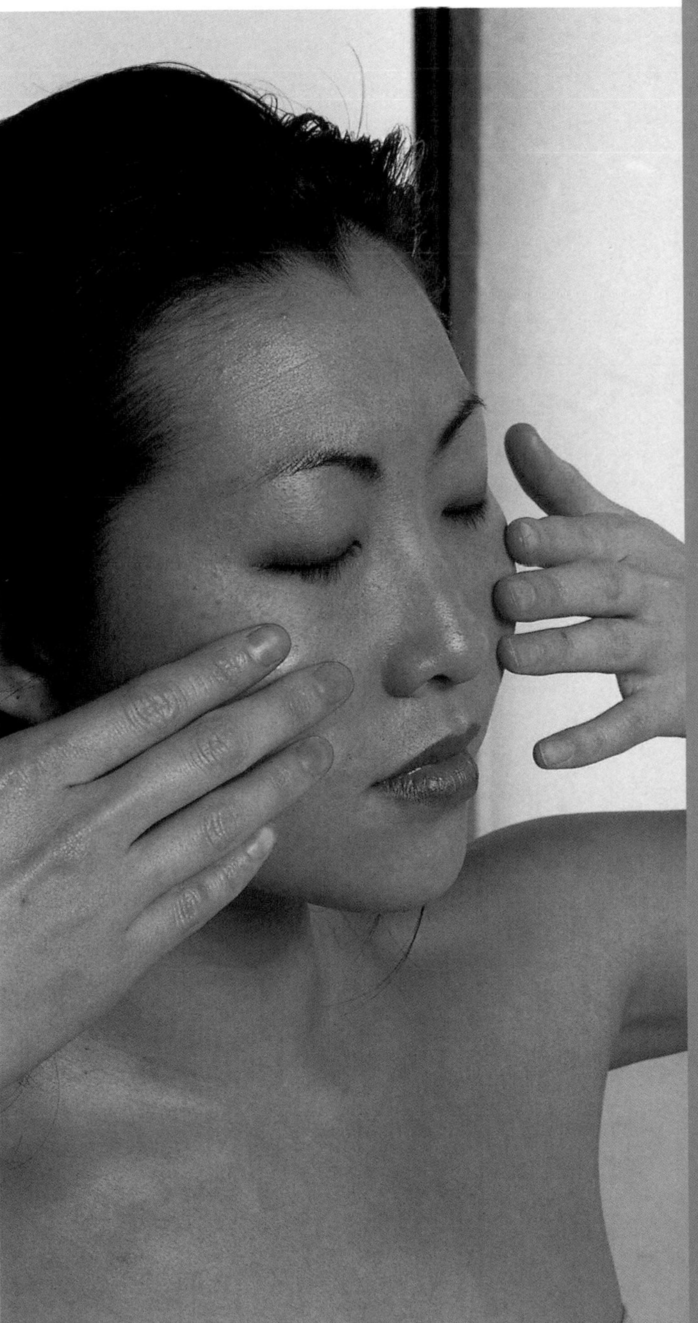

Personal preparation

Before giving an Indian head massage, make sure that you are prepared by running through the following checklist.

- Wear comfortable, loose-fitting clothes so that you can move around your partner easily. If you want to avoid becoming too warm, a loose-fitting, short-sleeved T-shirt, teamed with a pair of baggy trousers, is ideal. If you decide to use oil, choose practical fabrics that will wash easily in case you accidentally spill a small amount of oil on your clothes. Wear flat or low-heeled shoes or even none at all.
- Remove any jewellery, including your watch, to avoid scratching your partner.
- Make sure that your nails have been trimmed so that they won't dig into your partner.
- Wash your hands.
- Warm your hands.
- Shake your hands from the wrists to release any tension.
- Consciously relax yourself by breathing slowly and deeply. Focus on the treatment that you are about to give.

Preparing your partner

Before giving your partner an Indian head massage, you'll need to prepare him or her as follows.

- Ask your partner to remove any earrings, necklaces or body-piercing jewellery.
- If your partner wears spectacles, ask him or her to remove them.
- Brush through your partner's hair so that you won't pull on any tangles while you're giving the treatment.
- If your partner has long hair, use a hairclip or another type of hair accessory to tie it up while you are working on the neck, shoulders and upper back.
- Ensure that your partner is wearing appropriate clothing. If you are not using any oil, a loose-fitting T-shirt is ideal. If you are using oil, ask your partner to take off his or her top and then wrap a large towel or piece of natural fabric, such as cotton or silk, around his or her chest.
- Check for any contraindications or reasons why you shouldn't give your partner an Indian head massage (see pages 23 to 24).

Equipment and procedures

INDIAN HEAD MASSAGE is traditionally performed with the receiver seated. If your partner desires an even more relaxing treatment, however, he or she may lie down. Both positions have the same overall benefits.

Equipment needed if the receiver is seated

- An upright chair with quite a low back
- Pillows or cushions
- Towels
- Carrier oil and essential oils (optional)
- Crystals (optional)

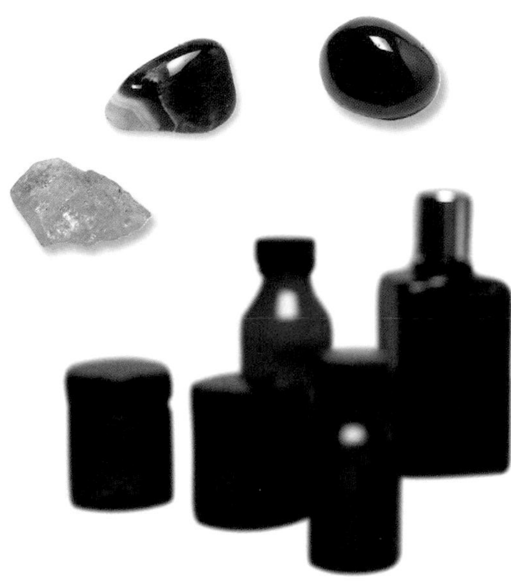

Equipment needed if the receiver is lying down

Either a massage couch or a duvet, futon, sleeping bag or one or two blankets with which to create a well-padded surface on the floor

- Pillows or cushions
- Towels
- Carrier oil and essential oils (optional)
- Crystals (optional)

Working with a seated partner

1 Select a chair for your partner to sit on that enables you to reach his or her scalp and shoulders comfortably without having to bend or strain.

2 Ask your partner to remove his or her shoes. Now seat your partner comfortably in the chair, ensuring that his or her legs aren't crossed and that their feet are resting on the ground.

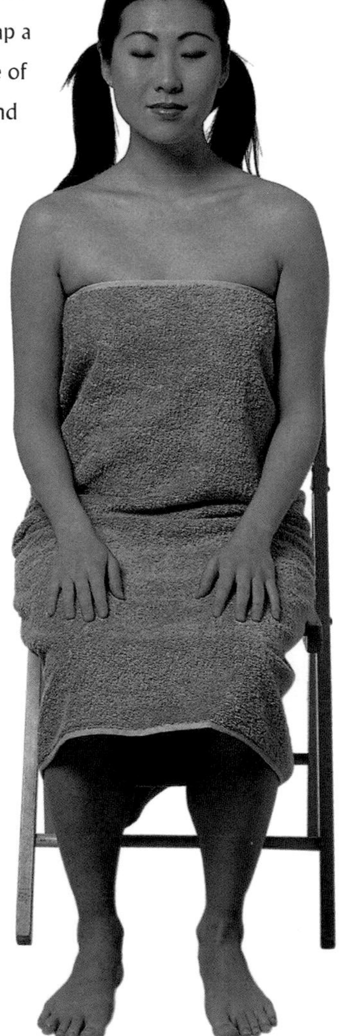

If you are using oil for your treatment, wrap a large towel or piece of natural fabric around your partner.

3 Place a pillow or cushion on your partner's lap and ask him or her to rest their hands lightly on it. You may like to give your partner a crystal to hold in each hand while you are working. Smooth, rounded stones are particularly suitable. Recommended crystals include:

- AMETHYST – clears negative and blocked energy;
- ANGELITE – bestows inner peace and angelic attunement;
- BLOODSTONE – gives courage, strength and stability;
- CLEAR QUARTZ, the 'master' healer – clears blockages and increases energy;
- GREEN CALCITE – balances the nerves;
- HAEMATITE – dispels negativity and stress and grounds the receiver at the end of a treatment;
- ROSE QUARTZ – heals the heart and bestows peace and tranquillity.

4 Stand squarely behind your partner, with your back held straight and your weight evenly distributed between both feet. Bend your knees slightly and keep your neck and shoulders relaxed. Try to maintain this good posture throughout the treatment.

Working with a partner who is lying down

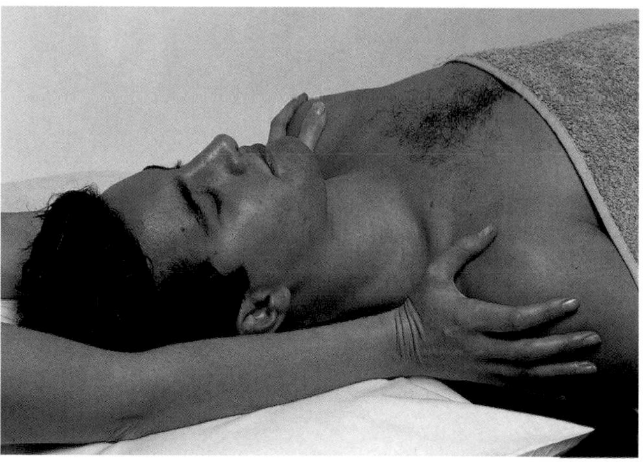

1 Create a firm, yet well-padded, surface by placing a duvet, futon, sleeping bag or one or two blankets on the floor. (If you possess a massage couch, this is ideal).

2 Ask your partner to lie on his or her back on the padded surface.

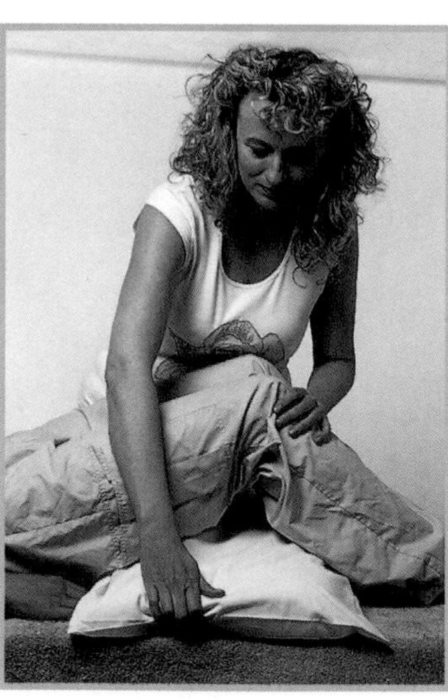

3 Place a pillow or cushion under your partner's head for comfort and one under the knees to take the pressure off the lower back.

4 Place a pillow or cushion close to your partner's head to kneel on so that you do not develop sore knees. Adjust your position so that you can comfortably reach under your partner's shoulders and around the back of the neck.

Contraindications or reasons for not giving an Indian head massage

INDIAN HEAD MASSAGE IS AN EXTREMELY SAFE AND GENTLE THERAPY. There are some instances, however, when a massage should either not be carried out or the advice of a doctor should be sought beforehand, as detailed below.

Instances when Indian head massage should not be given

- If the receiver has a high temperature or fever. This indicates that the body has raised its temperature to fight off infection and that it therefore does not need the burden of even more toxins to deal with.
- If the receiver has a thrombosis (blood clot). Giving a massage increases the risk that the blood clot could become detached, be carried to another part of the body and block the flow of blood to a vital organ.
- If the receiver has recently suffered a head or neck injury, for example a blow to the head or whiplash. A massage could exacerbate the condition and increase inflammation and pain.
- If the receiver has an infectious disease, such as chicken pox, measles, impetigo or scabies.
- If the receiver has a skin or scalp infection or infestation, such as head lice (Pediculosis) or ringworm of the scalp (Tinea capitis). Local areas of infection, as manifested by boils, carbuncles, conjunctivitis and styes, should also be avoided.
- If the receiver has any swellings or inflammation on the area to be massaged. Giving a massage would aggravate the inflammation.
- If the receiver is intoxicated. When the receiver is under the influence of alcohol, an increased flow of blood to the head could cause dizziness and nausea.
- If the receiver has had recent surgery involving the head and neck. Massaging recent scar tissue should always be avoided because it could cause pain and tissue damage, thereby interfering with the healing process.

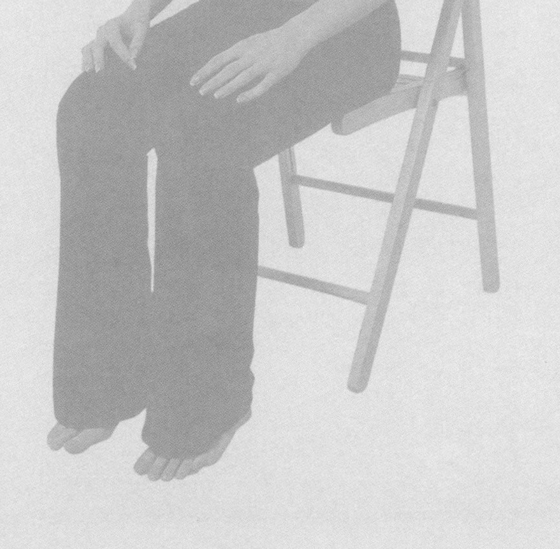

Instances when a doctor's advice should be sought or caution exercised

- If the receiver has any cuts, wounds, bruises, abrasions, bites, areas of sunburn, sensitive veins or areas of weeping eczema.
- If the receiver has any undiagnosed lumps and bumps. They may be cysts, but it is still advisable to have them checked out by a doctor before giving a massage.
- If the receiver has any suspicious moles. These should be checked by a doctor.
- If the receiver has very high or low blood pressure. Although massage is highly recommended for lowering blood pressure, patients taking medication for high blood pressure may feel dizzy and light-headed after the treatment. If so, advise them to get up slowly after the massage.
- If the receiver has a disorder of the nervous system, such as multiple sclerosis, Parkinson's disease or cerebral palsy. Only a gentle treatment should be given, which will help to reduce any spasms and rigidity.

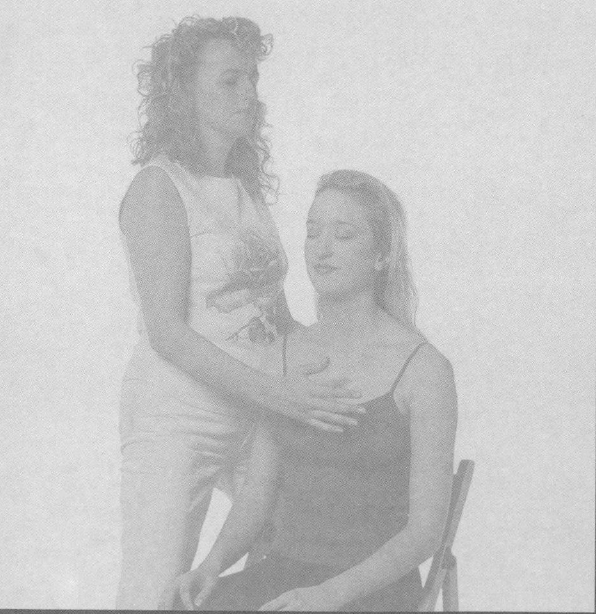

- If the receiver has epilepsy. Use gentle movements rather than stimulating ones.
- If the receiver has diabetes. Use gentle movements only and note that some diabetics may have a loss in sensory function and will therefore be unable to give feedback regarding pressure.
- If the receiver has osteoporosis (brittle bones). Use gentle movements only.
- If the receiver has a migraine. Do not carry out a treatment during an attack because this could make the symptoms worse. Indian head massage is excellent for preventing migraines, however, especially if they are stress-related.
- If the receiver is suffering from chronic fatigue. Use light movements only.
- If the receiver has cancer. Although massage is excellent for encouraging relaxation, avoid massaging any radiotherapy or tumour sites and areas of skin cancer.

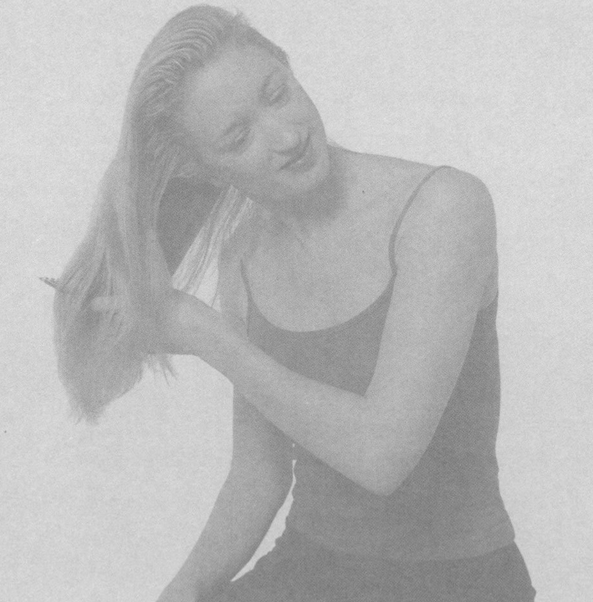

Oils and Indian Head Massage

ALTHOUGH CARRYING OUT a treatment without using an oil is acceptable, giving an Indian head massage with a lubricant will make the experience much more beneficial, pleasurable and relaxing for the receiver. Indeed, as we have already seen, oils are used for massaging both women and men in India.

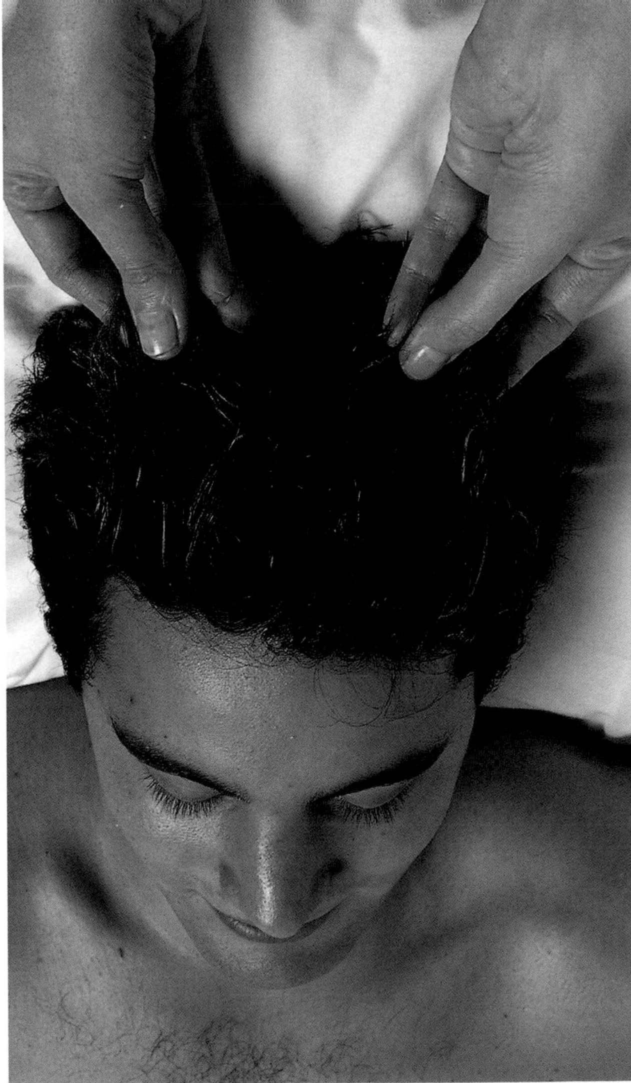

Types of carrier oil

A WIDE VARIETY OF CARRIER OILS is available to choose from. A pure, good-quality vegetable, nut or seed oil is recommended. The oil should ideally be cold-pressed (that is, no chemicals should have been involved in its making), unrefined and free of additives.

Such carrier oils contain vitamins, minerals and fatty acids and are therefore very therapeutic and nourishing for the skin and hair. Mineral oils, such as commercial baby oil, are not really suitable because they lack nutrients, are not easily absorbed and tend to clog the pores.

The oil that you select will probably be influenced by your personal preference, but try to be creative and to experiment with several different ones.

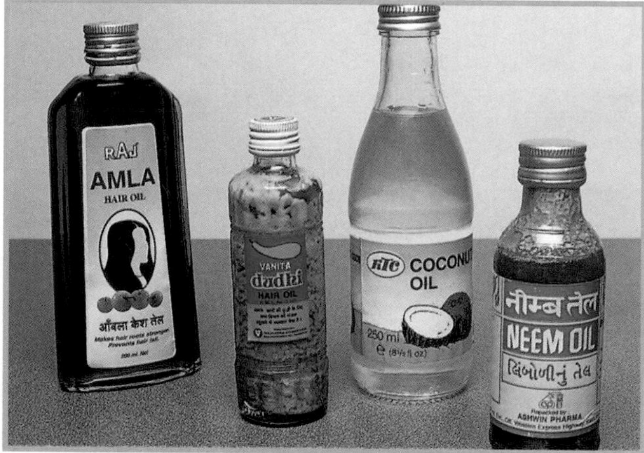

THE ADVANTAGES OF USING A CARRIER OIL ARE AS FOLLOWS:

- the oil enables your hands to glide smoothly over the skin and hair;
- the oil strengthens the hair;
- the oil promotes hair growth and decreases hair loss;
- the oil counteracts any dryness of the hair;
- the oil protects the hair from the drying effects of the sun;
- the oil makes the hair shiny and glossy;
- the oil nourishes and softens the scalp;
- the oil improves the condition of the scalp and skin by removing dead skin cells, eliminating waste products and improving the texture and tone of the skin and scalp.

In short, at the end of an Indian head massage using a carrier oil, the recipient's skin and hair will be glowing with health and vitality.

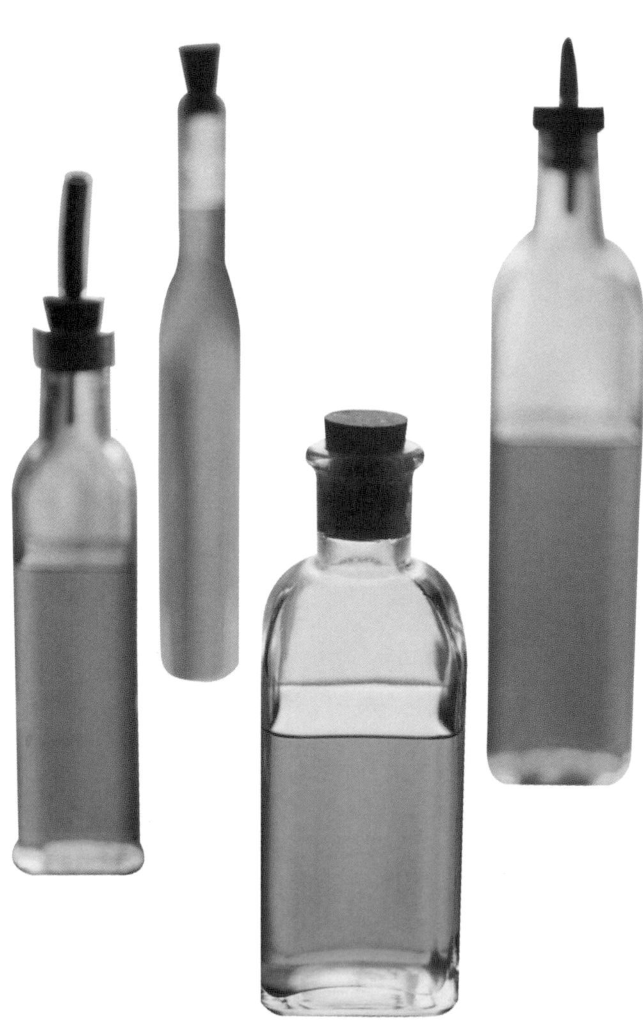

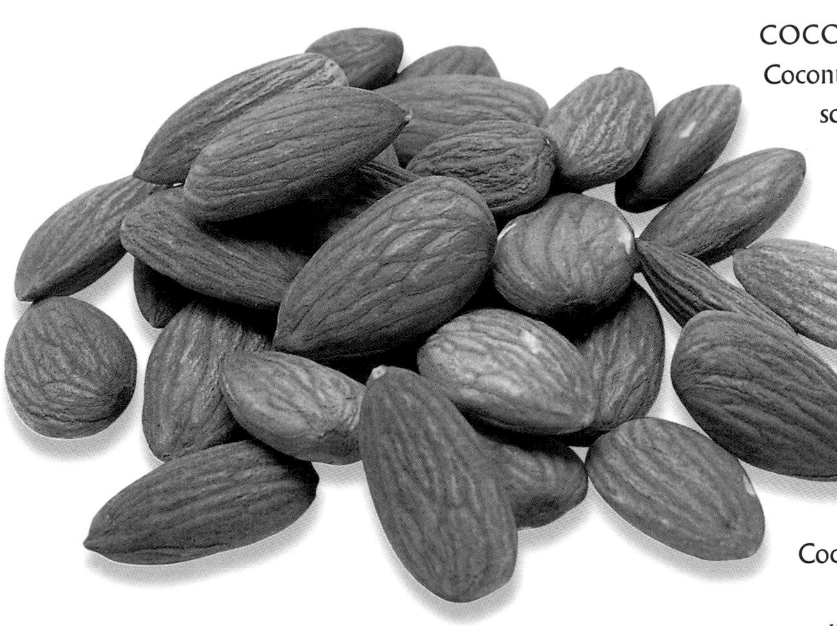

Popular carrier oils

ALMOND OIL (SWEET), *PRUNUS AMYGDALUS*

Sweet almond oil is both widely available and a popular carrier oil for use in massage. A versatile oil, it may be used to treat all skin and hair types. It is rich in vitamins, minerals and fatty acids and is a light oil that does not have a strong odour. Sweet almond oil is highly recommended for:

- all skin types;
- dry, sensitive or prematurely aged skin;
- dry hair and an itchy scalp.

Caution

Do not use bitter almond oil, which is highly toxic.

COCONUT OIL, *COCUS NUCIFERA*

Coconut oil is widely used in India, especially in the southern regions, for head massage, particularly in the spring and for women. A medium-to-light oil that is suitable for all skin and hair types, coconut oil has a distinctive aroma and is commonly used in the West by the cosmetics industry in soaps and tanning preparations, as well as in products for the hair and skin. (Because coconut oil is solid at room temperature, you may need to put it in a jug of hot water or near a radiator before using it.) Coconut oil is highly recommended for:

- all skin and hair types;
- dry, brittle hair;
- chemically treated hair;
- protecting the hair and skin from the sun's rays.

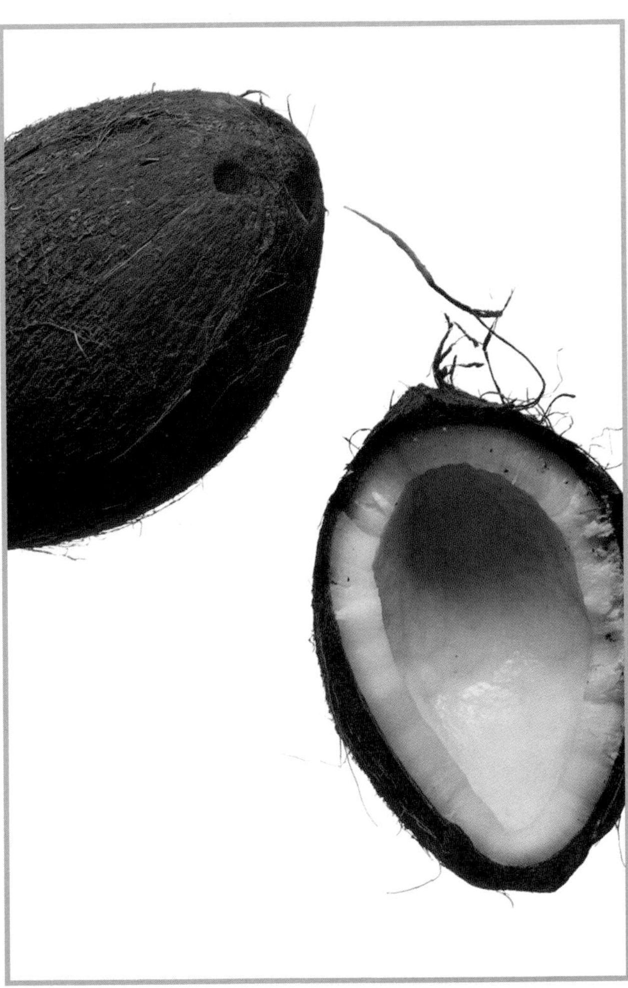

JOJOBA OIL, *SIMMONDSIA CHINENSIS*

A very balancing oil, jojoba makes an excellent treatment for all types of hair and skin. It also possesses anti-inflammatory properties, making it helpful when massaging people who suffer from arthritis or red, inflamed and irritated conditions of the scalp and skin. Jojoba nourishes, moisturises and has marvellous powers of penetration, and although it is expensive, in my opinion, the cost is worth it. Jojoba oil is highly recommended for:

- all types of hair and skin;
- damaged, brittle hair;
- dull hair;
- moisturising and rejuvenating the hair and skin.

MUSTARD OIL, *BRASSICA NIGRA*

One of the most popular oils for head massage in India, particularly in the north-west and for men, mustard oil is traditionally used in Ayurvedic medicine to counteract the cold quality of *kapha* types (see page 9). Because mustard oil is extremely warming and stimulating, it is a good choice in winter. It increases body heat, relieves pain, breaks down congestion and eases stiff muscles. Mustard oil is highly recommended for:

- warming or stimulating;
- use on men;
- relieving muscular tension and pain.

> **Caution**
> *Never use essential oil of mustard.*
> *Note that mustard oil may irritate sensitive skin.*
> *Do not use mustard oil on sensitive scalps.*

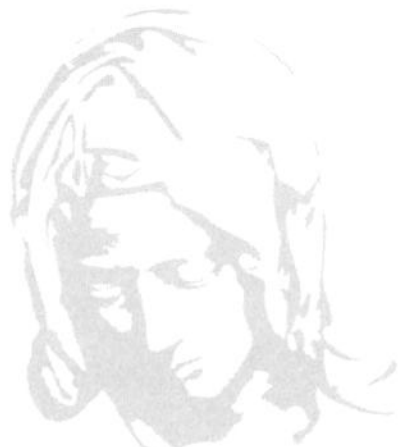

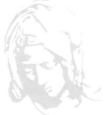

OLIVE OIL, *OLEA EUROPAEA*

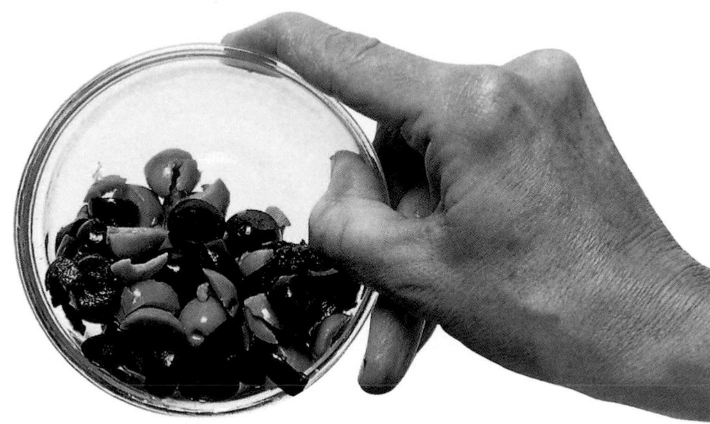

Traditionally used over the centuries for cooking and healing, olive oil is widely available in the Western world. In India, this rather strong-smelling oil is used especially in the summer. Only extra virgin olive oil should be used for massage, and because you may find this green, viscous liquid a little heavy, you may prefer to combine it with a less viscous oil, such as sweet almond oil, in a fifty-fifty mixture. Olive oil is highly recommended for:

- dry and brittle hair and dry skin;
- inflamed skin and scalps.

SESAME OIL, *SESAMUM INDICUM*

Sesame oil, which is widely used in Ayurvedic medicine, is possibly the most popular of the carrier oils used for hair massage in India. It is rich in vitamins and minerals, especially iron, phosphorus, calcium, vitamin E and sesamol. Although it may be used for all types of skin and hair, sesame oil has a nutty aroma, which some Westerners find off-putting. Sesame oil is highly recommended for:

- preventing the hair from turning grey;
- dry skin and hair;
- eczema and psoriasis;
- protecting the hair and skin from the sun's rays.

> **Caution**
> *Sesame oil may irritate highly sensitive skin.*

Other carrier oils

The following carrier oils may also be used for Indian head massage.

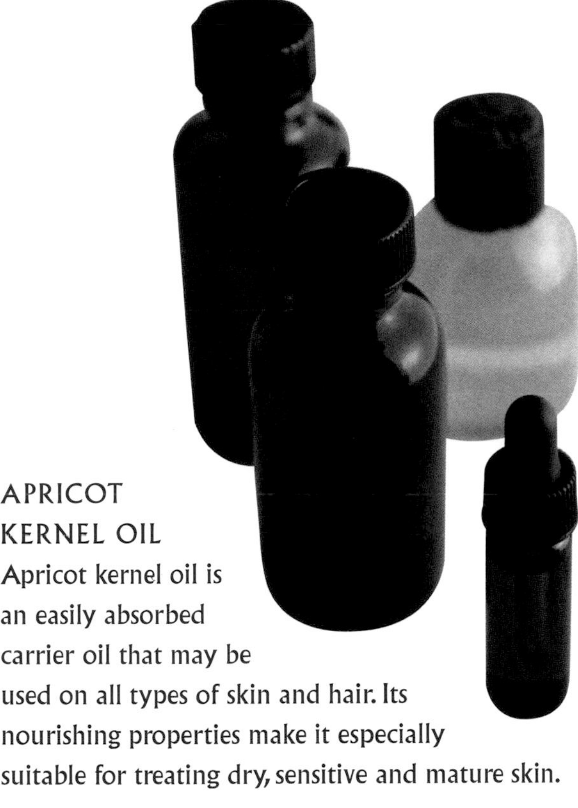

APRICOT KERNEL OIL

Apricot kernel oil is an easily absorbed carrier oil that may be used on all types of skin and hair. Its nourishing properties make it especially suitable for treating dry, sensitive and mature skin.

GRAPESEED OIL

Grapeseed oil is an odourless, colourless carrier oil. Light in texture, it may be used for all types of hair and skin.

PEACH KERNEL OIL

Peach kernel oil has very similar properties to sweet almond oil (see page 27) and apricot kernel oil (see above). It is particularly useful for treating dry and mature skin.

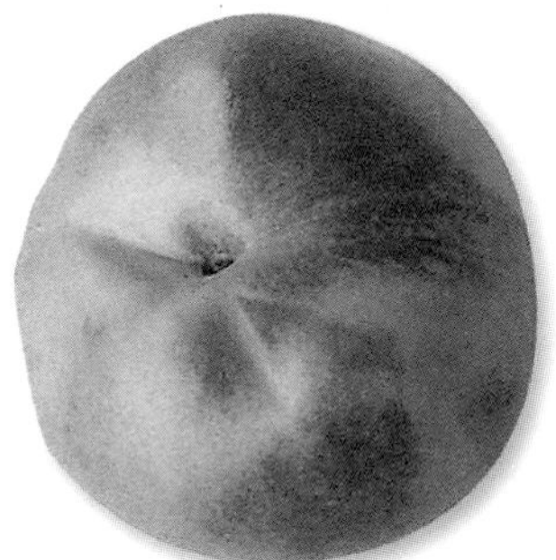

PUMPKIN SEED OIL

A very nourishing oil, pumpkin-seed oil is useful for treating dry and brittle hair.

SAFFLOWER OIL

The use of safflower oil is indicated if the receiver suffers from inflammation and poor circulation.

SUNFLOWER OIL

Suitable for all skin types, sunflower oil has a light texture and is particularly helpful when massaging skin that is prone to inflammation and rashes.

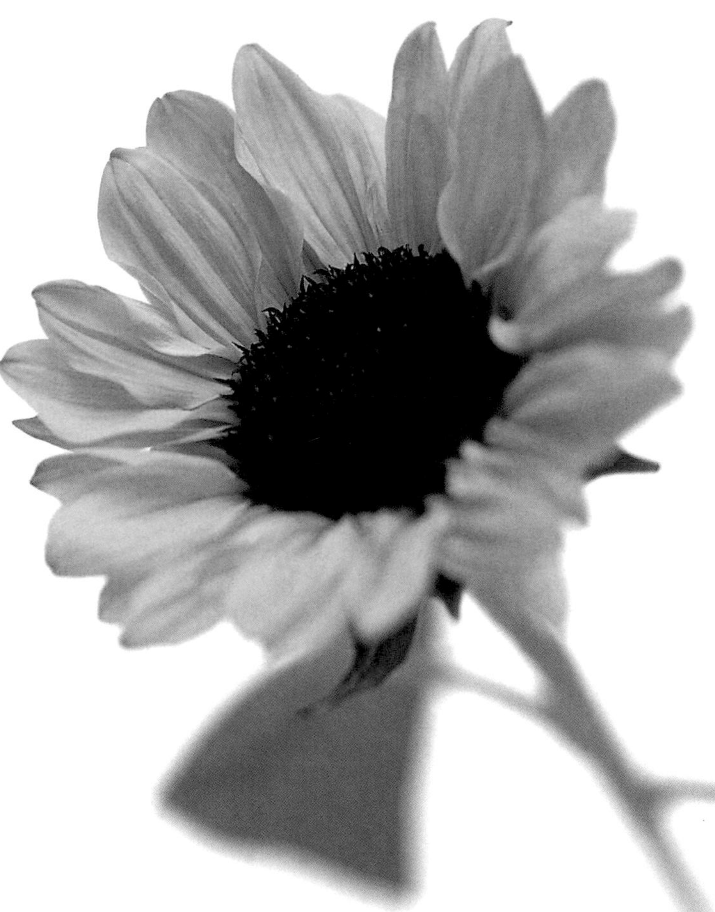

WHEATGERM OIL

Due to its high vitamin E content, wheatgerm oil is usually added to another carrier oil in a dilution of up to ten per cent to prolong the life of a blend. This oil is excellent for soothing dry, cracked, itchy and flaky skin and scalps.

More unusual Indian massage oils

Although the following oils are commonly used in India for head massage, they are not so readily available in the West. They may, however, be found in some traditional Indian supermarkets.

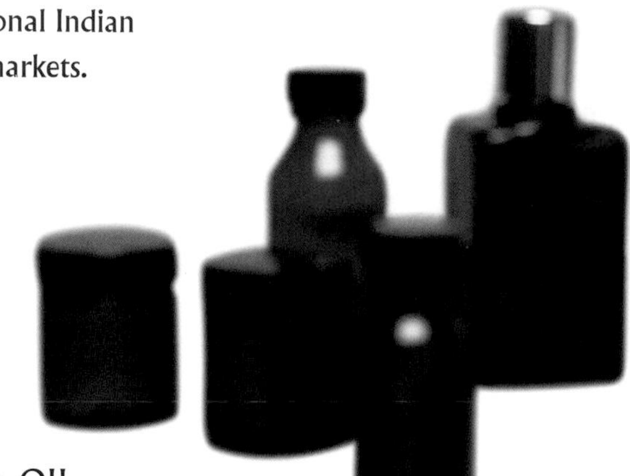

AMLA OIL

Amla oil is prepared from dried amla berries that have been soaked in coconut oil for several days. The amla fruit is one of the richest natural sources of vitamin C and the oil is said to boost hair growth and to prevent premature greying. Amla oil is also used as a general tonic for improving a person's well-being.

BHRINGARAJ OIL

Bhringaraj oil is excellent for promoting the growth and health of the hair. Said to prevent hair loss and to reverse greying, it is believed to prevent ageing in general and to rejuvenate not only the hair, but also the teeth, bones, memory, sight and hearing. Bhringaraj also promotes deep sleep and improves the complexion. It is often mixed with coconut, almond, olive or sesame oil, or a combination of these oils, to treat thick, dark hair.

BRAHMI OIL

Brahmi oil is popular for use in head and scalp massages in India. Not only does brahmi oil encourage hair growth, but it also promotes intelligence, improves the memory and dispels mental fatigue. It is an excellent tonic for the nerves, too.

NEEM OIL

Neem oil is commonly used in India for alleviating all sorts of skin disorders, including fungal conditions, acne, dry skin, wounds, abrasions and rashes.

SHIKAKAI OIL

Shikakai oil is excellent for promoting hair growth and for soothing a dry, itchy scalp. In addition, it is thought to prevent dandruff.

RECOMMENDED CARRIER OILS FOR THE *DOSHAS*

Certain carrier oils are recommended for treating each of the three *dosha* types, as listed below.

FOR THE *VATA* CONSTITUTION (COOL, DRY AND NERVOUS)

- *almond oil*
- *amla oil*
- *bala oil*
- *neem oil*
- *olive oil*
- *sesame oil*
- *wheatgerm oil*

FOR THE *PITTA* CONSTITUTION (HOT, OILY AND PRONE TO RASHES, INFLAMMATION OR BLEMISHES)

- *almond oil*
- *coconut oil*
- *jojoba oil*
- *pumpkin-seed oil*
- *sesame oil*
- *sunflower oil*

FOR THE *KAPHA* CONSTITUTION (COOL, HEAVY AND SLOW)

- *mustard oil*
- *neem oil*
- *safflower oil*
- *sesame oil*

Essential oils

ESSENTIAL OILS can both enhance an Indian head massage and promote and preserve the natural beauty of the hair and skin. They can be used to treat specific hair and skin conditions, too.

It is important to remember that essential oils must never be used neat as they are so highly concentrated and they should always be diluted by, or blended with, a suitable carrier oil (see pages 26 to 29 for descriptions of the best-known carrier oils).

Blending oils

Blending an essential oil with a carrier oil is a very simple, yet exciting, process. Because essential oils can damage varnished or plastic surfaces, always mix your oils on a worktop that is easily washable.

WHAT YOU WILL NEED

- A small glass bowl or a coloured glass bottle
- Carrier oils(s)
- Essential oil(s) – choose no more than three

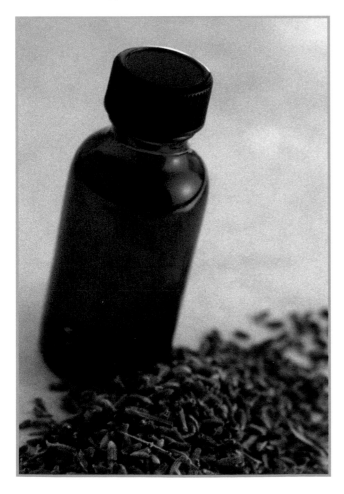

1 Measure out 10ml (2 teaspoons) of the carrier oil into the bowl or bottle.

2 Add three drops of the essential oil. (If you have selected three different essential oils, add only one drop of each.)

3 If you are using a bowl, mix the oils together well; if you are using a bottle, shake it gently.

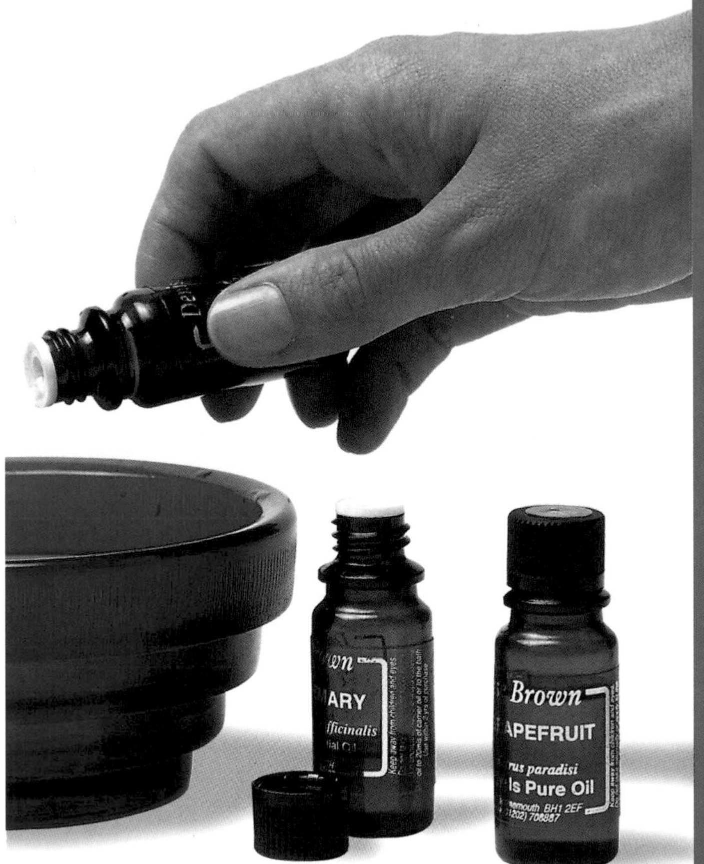

Storing blends of oil

If you hit on a blend of oils that you want to use on a regular basis, you will need to store it in an amber-coloured glass bottle. These are available in various sizes, but you will probably find the 50ml or 100ml sizes the most appropriate for your needs. To prolong the life of your blend, make sure that you include a teaspoon of wheatgerm carrier oil. It's important to store your blend in a cool, dry, dark place because essential oils are adversely affected by sunlight, warm temperatures, air and moisture. If stored properly, a blend should keep for three to six months.

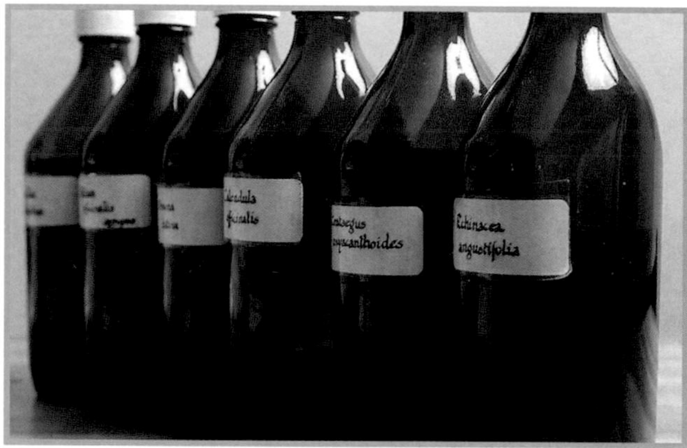

You can also blend your oils into creams or lotions. For the best results, use a non-mineral, organic, lanolin-free base (see the useful addresses section on page 112 for suppliers). The essential oil should again be diluted, in the proportion of 3 drops of essential oil to 10gm cream. See the box below for further dilution proportions.

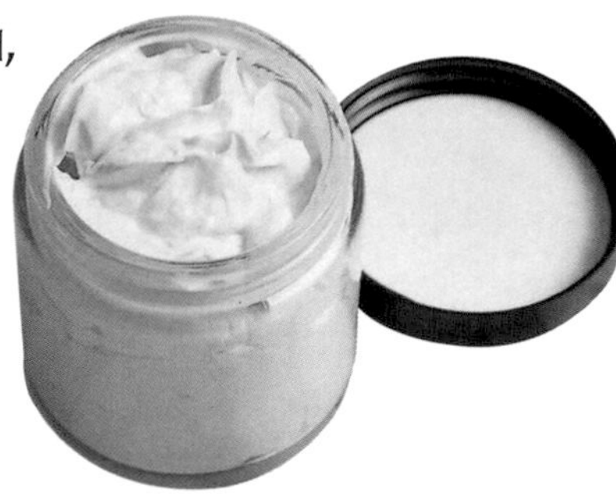

DILUTIONS

3 drops of essential oil to 10ml of carrier oil
6 drops of essential oil to 20ml of carrier oil
15 drops of essential oil to 50ml of carrier oil
30 drops of essential oil to 100ml of carrier oil

Introducing a selection of essential oils

There are hundreds of essential oils, so, to avoid confusion, as well as for the sake of simplicity and cost, I will introduce you to only a small selection of the ones that I recommend for treating various conditions of the hair and skin.

OILS FOR DRY HAIR AND SKIN

Dry hair and skin are caused by underactive sebaceous glands that are not producing enough sebum. They can also be caused by overexposure to the sun, chemical treatments, heated hair appliances and the overuse of strong shampoo. The essential and carrier oils that I've therefore recommended are designed to activate the sebaceous glands, relieve dryness and ultimately make the hair glossy and shiny.
[X25, coconut – to come]

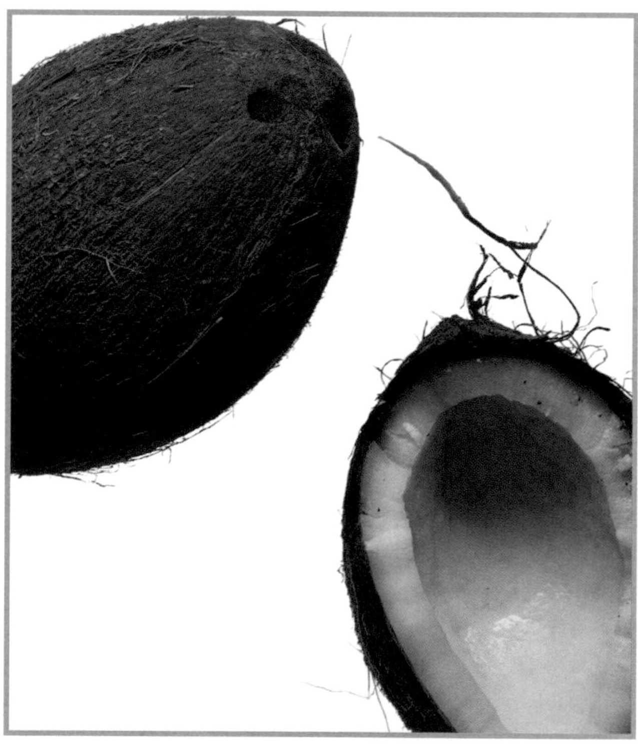

Suggested essential oils
Carrot seed, chamomile, frankincense, geranium, lavender, neroli, rose, sandalwood or ylang ylang.

Suggested carrier oils
Sweet almond, apricot kernel, avocado, coconut, jojoba, olive, peach kernel, sesame or wheatgerm.

OILS FOR OILY HAIR AND SKIN

Oily hair and skin are due to the overactivity of the sebaceous glands. Particularly common during puberty, these conditions can be exacerbated by stress and a poor diet.

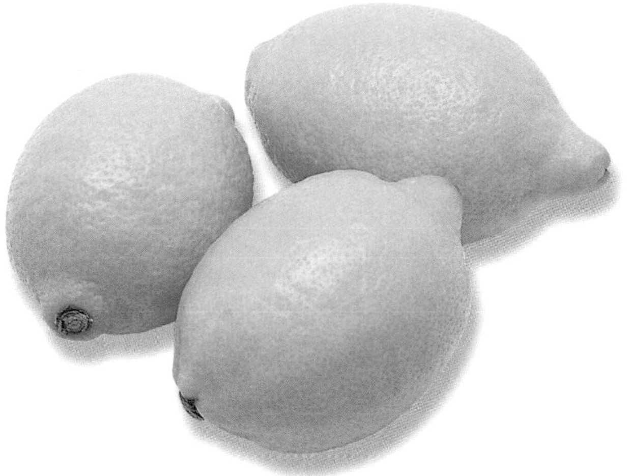

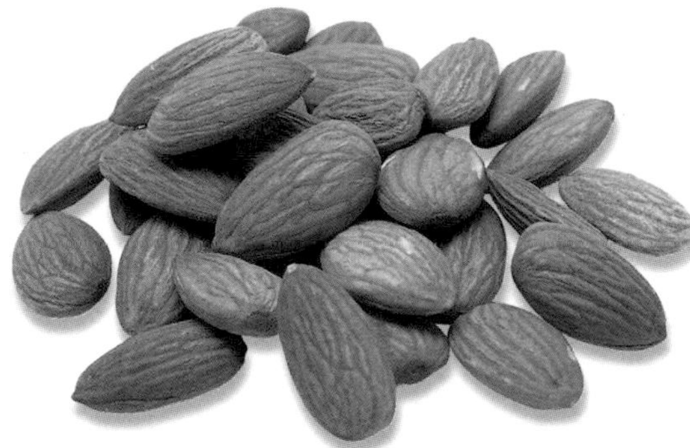

Suggested essential oils

Bergamot, cedarwood, cypress, geranium, juniper, lemon or rosemary.

Suggested carrier oils

Sweet almond, apricot kernel, peach kernel or jojoba.

OILS FOR NORMAL HAIR AND SKIN

Normal hair should be glossy and strong, while normal skin should be blemish-free and glowing with health. However, both need to be nurtured if their health is to be maintained.

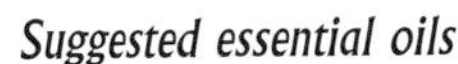

Suggested essential oils

Carrot seed, chamomile, geranium, lavender, rosemary or rosewood.

Colour-enhancing essential oils

- chamomile is excellent for fair hair;
- carrot seed is excellent for red hair;
- rosemary and rosewood are excellent for dark hair.

Suggested carrier oils

Sweet almond, apricot kernel, jojoba or peach kernel.

OILS FOR SENSITIVE SKIN AND SCALPS

Sensitive skin and scalps are often caused by the chemicals in shampoos, dyes and perming solutions. The wrong sort of diet and stress can also make the skin hypersensitive.

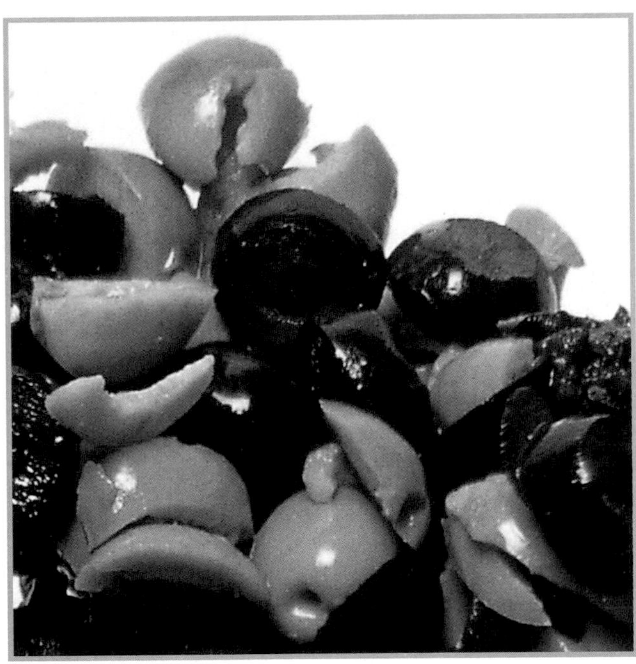

Suggested essential oils

Chamomile, lavender, neroli or rose.

Suggested carrier oils

Sweet almond, apricot kernel, evening primrose, olive or jojoba.

OILS FOR HAIR LOSS

Hair loss can either be a genetic condition or caused by hormonal imbalances. High stress levels, poor diet, tension within the scalp and chemical treatments can also cause hair loss.

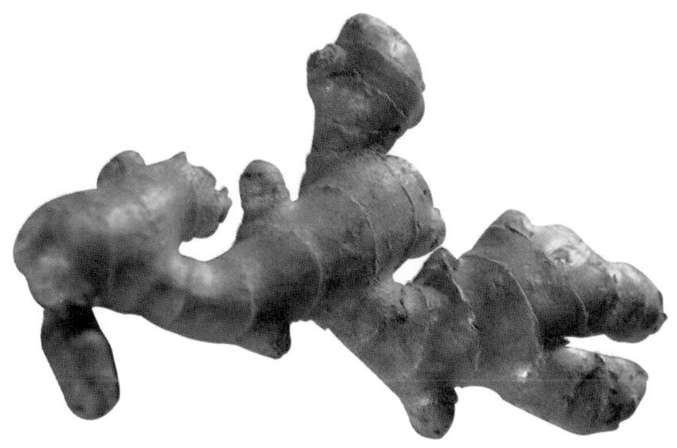

Suggested essential oils

Cedarwood, clary sage, cypress, frankincense, geranium, ginger or rosemary.

Suggested carrier oils

Sweet almond, jojoba, mustard, olive or sesame.

OILS FOR DANDRUFF

It is natural for the scalp to shed dead skin cells, but if the rate of shedding is so excessive that the cells cannot be removed by washing, dandruff may be diagnosed. Dry dandruff is characterised by dry, white flakes, whereas oily dandruff is characterised by yellowish, sticky flakes.

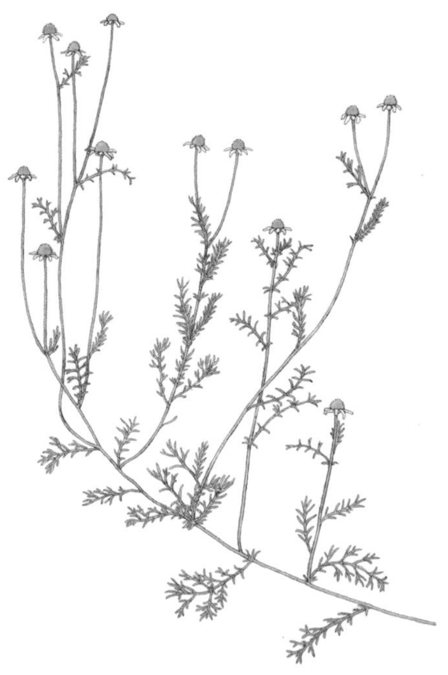

Suggested essential oils

Carrot seed, cedarwood, chamomile, patchouli or sandalwood.

Suggested carrier oils

Sweet almond, coconut, jojoba, olive or wheatgerm.

OILS FOR HEAD LICE

Children are particularly prone to catching head lice and are likely to have them at least once during their school career. Regular massage with essential oils can help to prevent the problem from occurring.

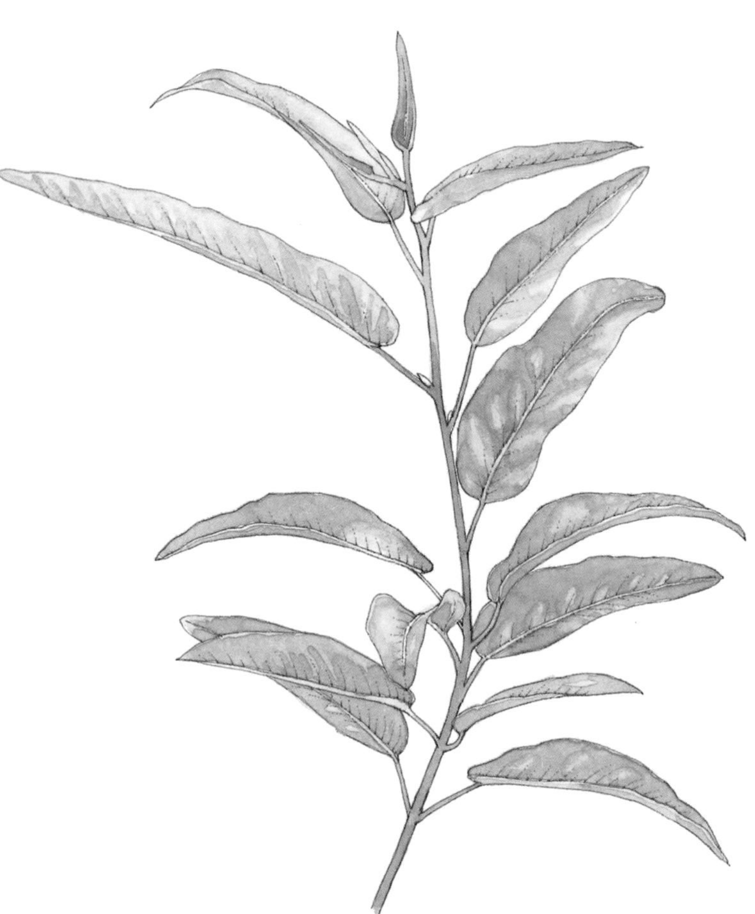

Suggested essential oils

Bergamot, eucalyptus, geranium, lavender, lemon, rosemary or tea tree.

Suggested carrier oils

Sweet almond, jojoba, apricot kernel or peach kernel.

Basic Techniques for Indian Head Massage

THIS CHAPTER WILL FAMILIARISE YOU with the basic movements used in Indian head massage. Once you have mastered them, you can create your own strokes and develop a unique style.

Do not worry if you feel clumsy at first, because massage is an instinctive therapy. We all have a natural ability to give a massage, and you will be amazed by how easily you master the movements and, with practice, how flowing your massage strokes will become.

Practice the massage techniques with your partner in the sitting position. Although you don't have to use oil, applying a lubricant will make it easier for your hands to guide smoothly and comfortably over the skin. If you are using it, place your oil within easy reach (perhaps in a flip-top bottle or, if you are working with a blend of oils, in a small bowl), ideally on a small table or stool beside you.

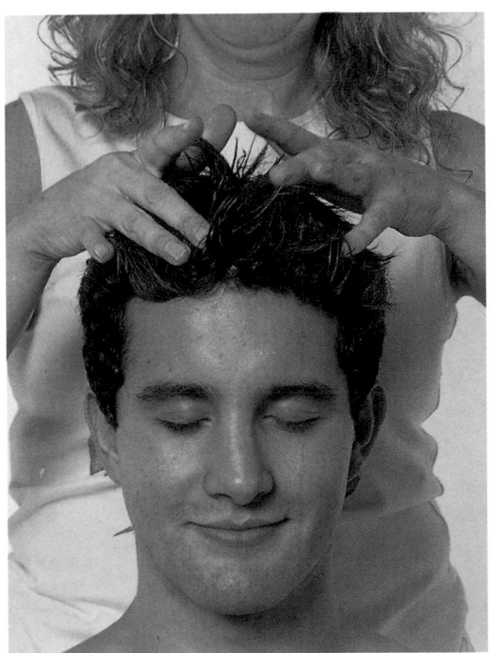

Effleurage or stroking

EFFLEURAGE IS A RHYTHMIC, stroking movement that is usually performed either with the palm of one hand or the palms of both. This technique is always performed at the beginning and at the end of a massage. It is also used as a link between movements.

An Indian head massage consists of a mixture of gentle, slow stroking movements and brisk, energetic stroking movements. Slow, soft stroking, which is used to relax the body and mind, is very soporific and will enable your partner to forget the stresses and strains of everyday life. Brisk stroking, on the other hand, will refresh and revitalise and dispel feelings of lethargy and weariness.

Because effleurage is performed at the beginning of the treatment, it helps your partner to become accustomed to the feel of your hands. As you effleurage, allow your hands gently to mould to the contours of your partner's body, and a relationship of trust will be established as the receiver gently melts into your hands. Stroking is a very pleasurable technique, to give, as well as to receive.

THE BENEFITS OF EFFLEURAGE

Effleurage is beneficial because it:

- *spreads the oil;*
- *accustoms your partner to the feel of your hands;*
- *establishes a sense of trust;*
- *links movements together;*
- *soothes the sensory nerve endings through slow stroking, inducing a deep sense of relaxation;*
- *relaxes tense muscles;*
- *warms the area of skin, as fresh blood is brought to the surface;*
- *assists the removal of dead skin cells, thus encouraging new cell growth;*
- *stimulates the sebaceous glands so that the skin is moisturised;*
- *stimulates the sweat glands to cleanse the skin;*
- *encourages the elimination of toxins, as the lymphatic system is stimulated;*
- *invigorates, energises and stimulates through brisk stroking, dispelling lethargy and fatigue;*
- *prepares the body for the deeper massage movements that are to follow.*

Practice 1

Circular effleurage around the shoulder blades

Position yourself squarely behind the receiver, making sure that he or she is relaxed and comfortable and that their legs are uncrossed. If you are using oil, having first ensured that it is within easy reach, pour a small amount on to the palm of one hand and then rub your hands together to warm the oil.

1 Relax your hands and place them on the receiver's upper back, positioning a hand on either side of the spine, with your fingers facing upwards.

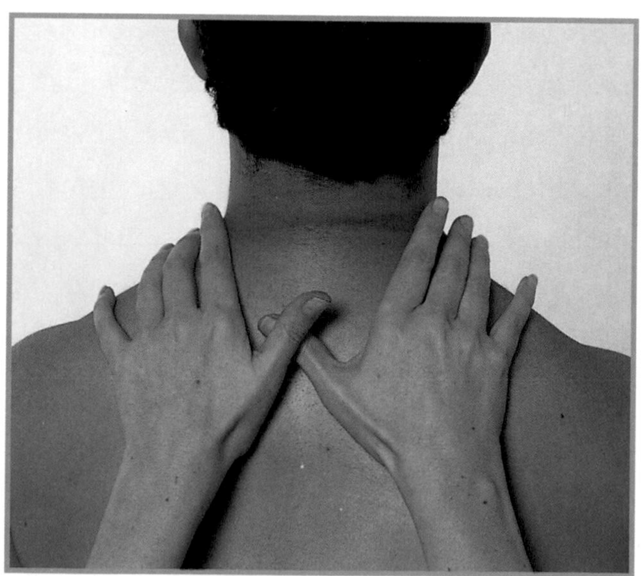

2 Using both hands simultaneously, perform large, stroking movements in a circular direction around the shoulder blades (scapulae). Experiment with different pressures and try using both firm and light touches. Ask your partner which he or she prefers. To exert firmer pressure, place one hand on top of the other and circle each shoulder blade individually.

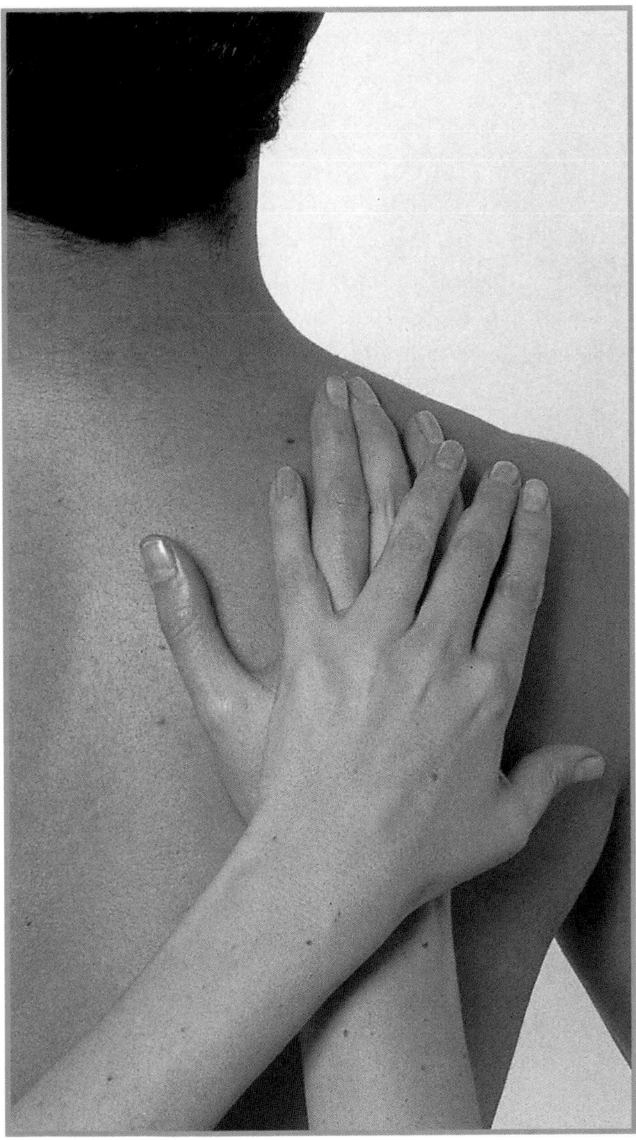

Practice 2

Stroking the head and shoulders

Stand behind the receiver and rest the palms of your hands very gently on the top of their head.

1 Using a gentle touch, slowly stroke down your partner's head, allowing the movement to continue down the neck and across the top of the shoulders. With a feather-light touch, return your hands to the top of your partner's head. Close your eyes to heighten your sensitivity and feel how deeply relaxed your partner is becoming.

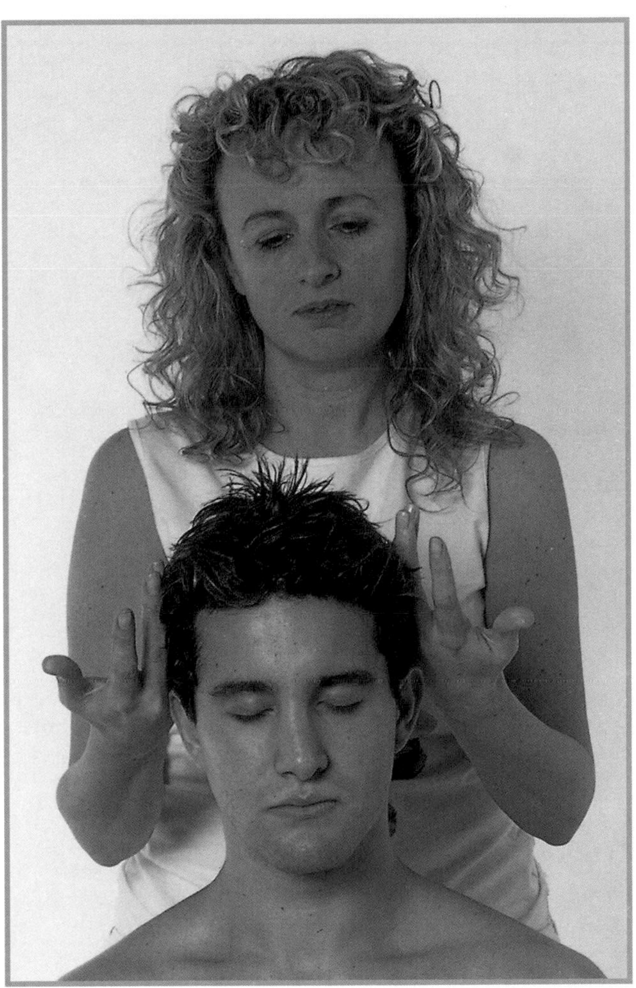

2 Now perform the same stroking movements using the backs and sides of both of your hands instead of your palms. Feel the difference in the quality of the movements. Experiment, too, with using only the pads of several fingers.

3 You may also stroke using only one hand. To do this, gently rest the palm of one hand on top of your partner's head and use the palm and back of your other hand gently to stroke down the head and neck.

Petrissage or kneading or squeezing

PETRISSAGE ALLOWS YOU TO WORK DEEPLY on the muscles and is therefore performed on the fleshy areas of the body. The action is rather like kneading dough: soft tissue is picked up, squeezed and then released. The muscle may also be rolled.

The palms of the hands can be used to perform petrissage, as well as the fleshy pads of the fingers and thumbs, although in an Indian head massage the fingers and thumbs are mostly employed.

THE BENEFITS OF PETRISSAGE

Petrissage is beneficial because:

- *the deeper tissues are worked on;*
- *waste products are eliminated;*
- *blood flow is increased so that fresh nutrients are brought to the area of skin;*
- *knots and nodules of tension are loosened and broken down;*
- *muscle spasm is released;*
- *muscle tone is improved;*
- *fatty deposits are broken down;*
- *the sebaceous glands are stimulated;*
- *it induces a sense of well-being as tension is released.*

Practice 1

Picking up and squeezing the shoulder muscle

Place the palm of each hand on top of each of your partner's shoulders, with your thumbs at the back and your fingers over the top of the shoulders.

1 Grasp the muscle firmly with both hands, pick it up to separate it from the underlying structure, squeeze and then release it. It should feel as though you have suction pads on the palms of your hands. Make sure that you are not pinching the receiver and thereby causing discomfort.

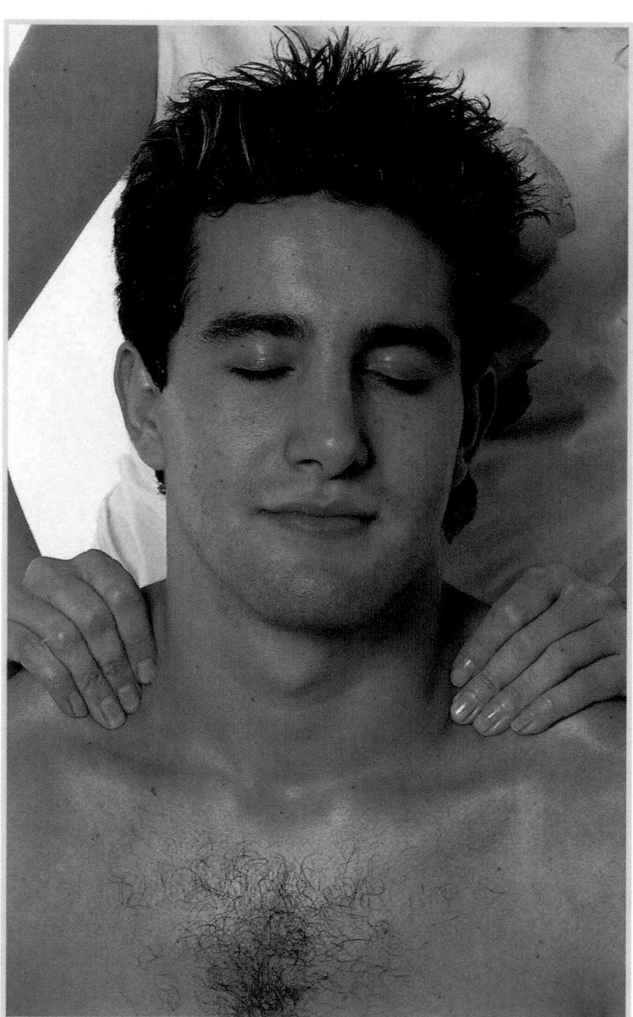

2 Place the palms of both of your hands on one of your partner's shoulders, squeeze and then release the tissues. Not only should you be able to feel the tissue moving, but also knots and nodules of tension.

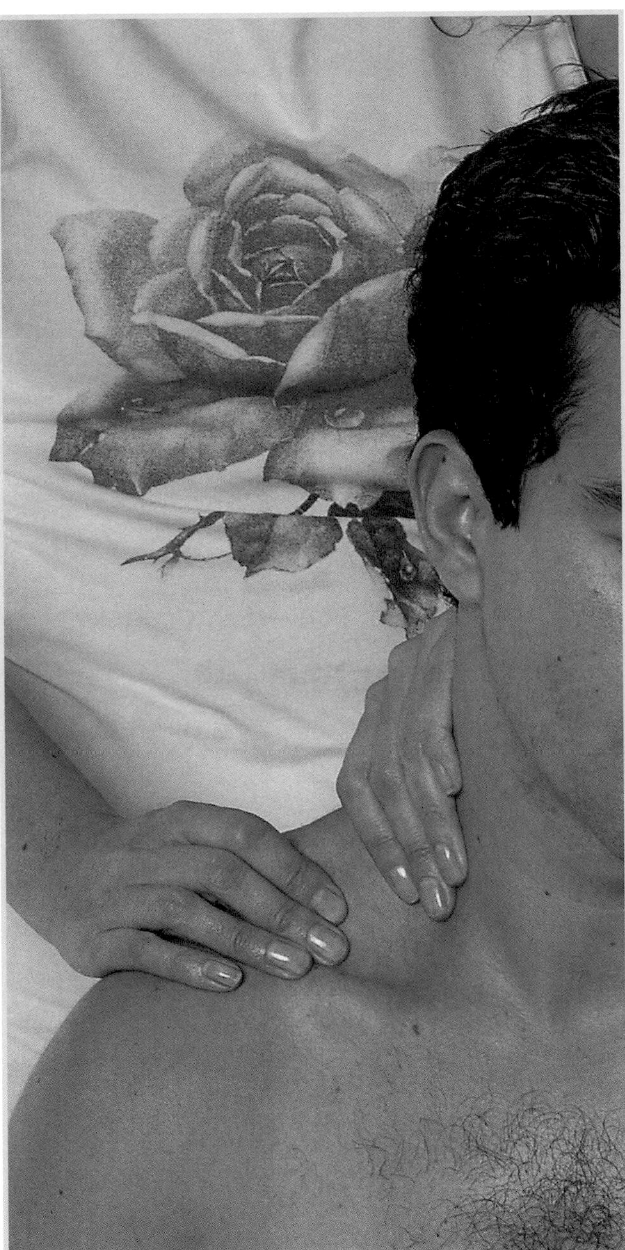

Practice 2

Picking up and squeezing the upper arm muscles

Place the palms of your hands on the top of each of the receiver's arms.

1 Working from the top of the arms to the elbows, firmly squeeze and release the tissues.

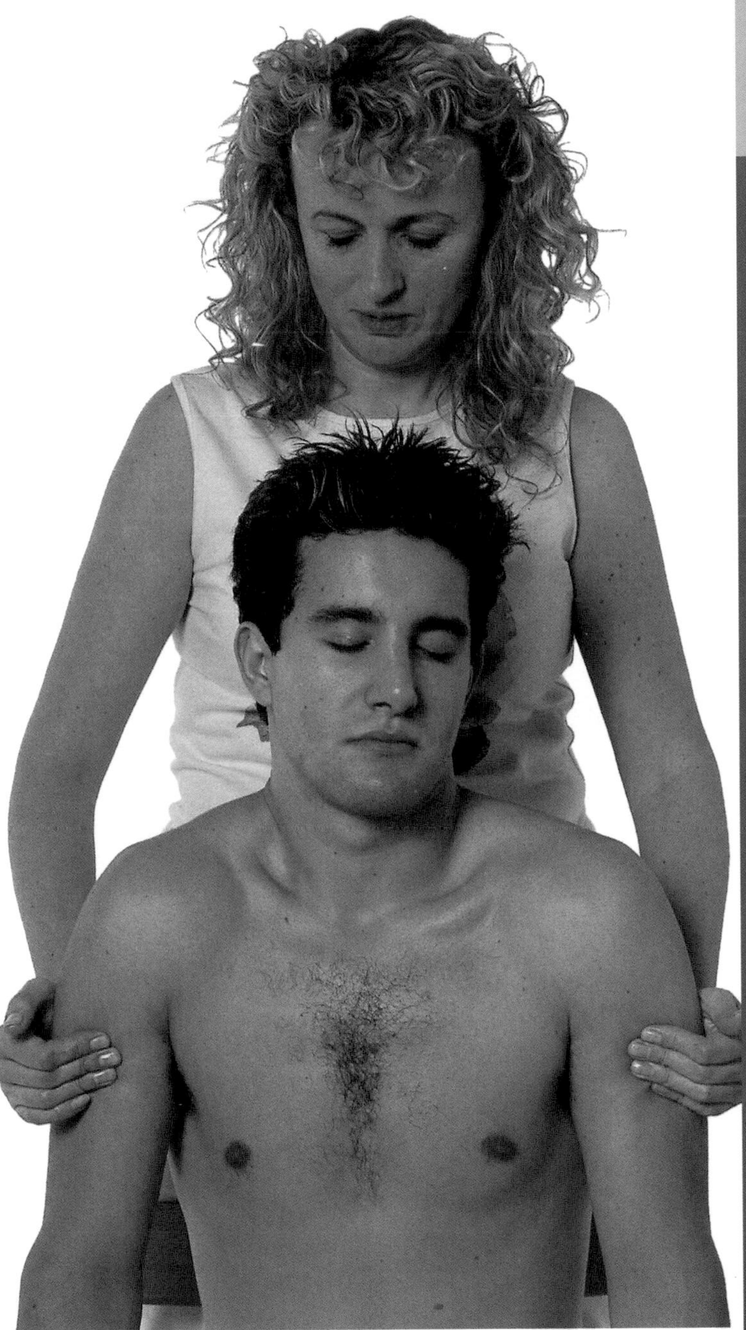

2 As well as the sides, make sure that you cover both the front and the back of the arms.

3 Now allow both hands to glide gently back to their starting position.

Practice 3

Picking up and rolling the shoulder muscles

THUMB PUSHES

1 Place the palms of your hands on the edge of each of the receiver's shoulders, with your thumbs at the back, just above the shoulder blades, and your fingers in front of the shoulders. Pushing your thumbs forwards, towards your fingers, pick up and squeeze as much flesh as you can. (see below)

2 Move your hands to the middle of the receiver's shoulders and repeat the action. Now repeat the action again near the neck.

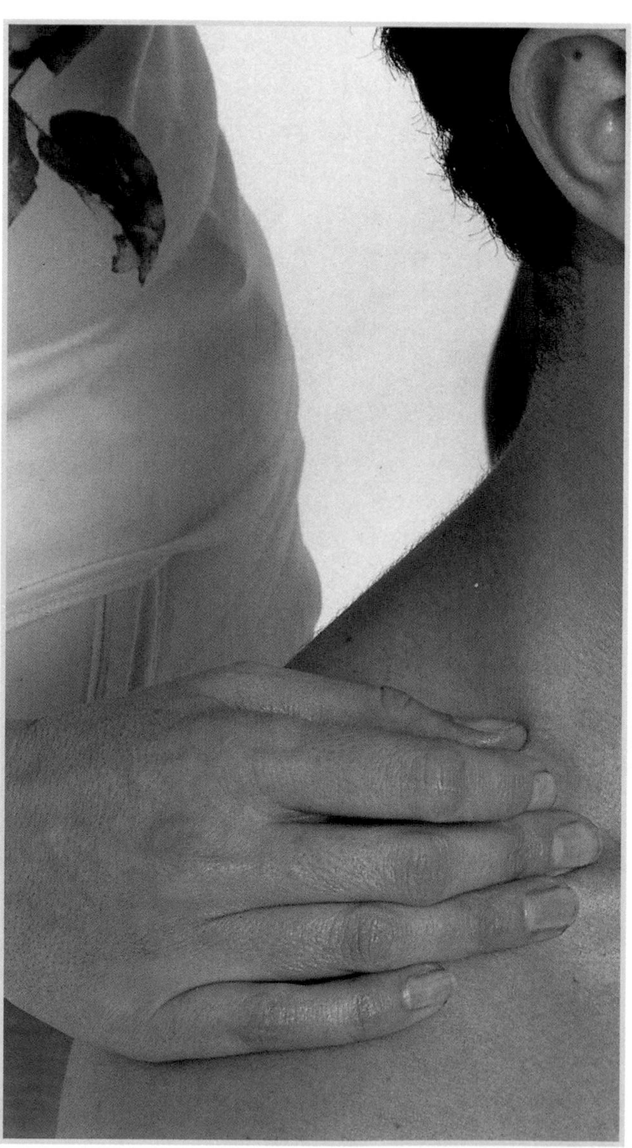

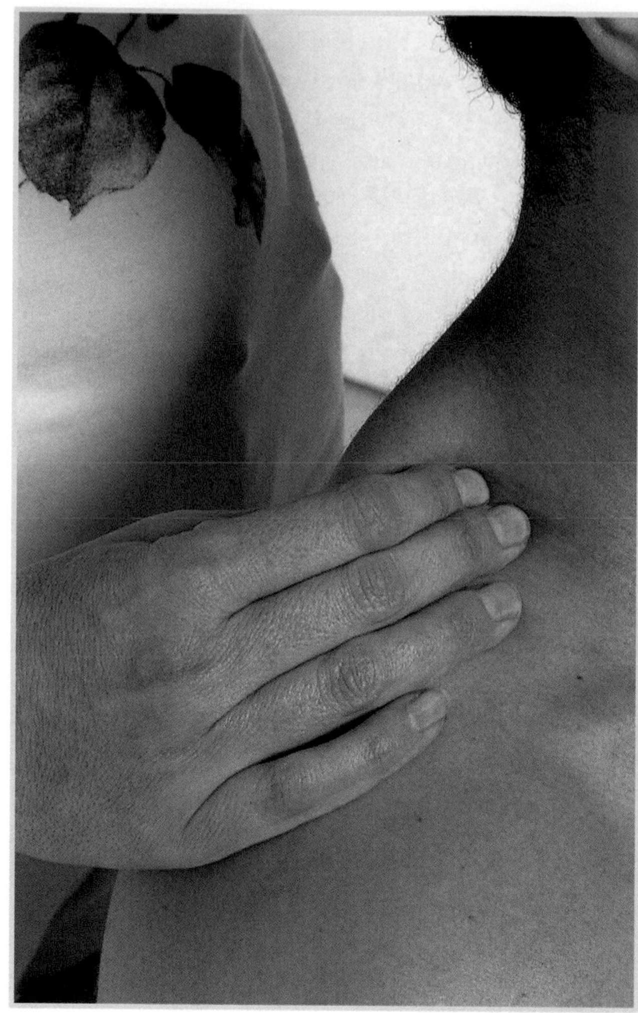

FINGER PULLS

1 Position your hands as described in step 1 of the thumb pushes, above, but instead of pushing your thumbs over the shoulder muscles, pull back the muscles by pulling your fingers towards your thumbs. (see above)

2 Move your hands to the middle of the receiver's shoulders and repeat the action. Now repeat the action again near the neck.

Practice 4

Squeezing and rolling the shoulder muscles

1 Rest the palms of your hands on top of each of the recipient's shoulders, with your fingers and thumbs at the front.

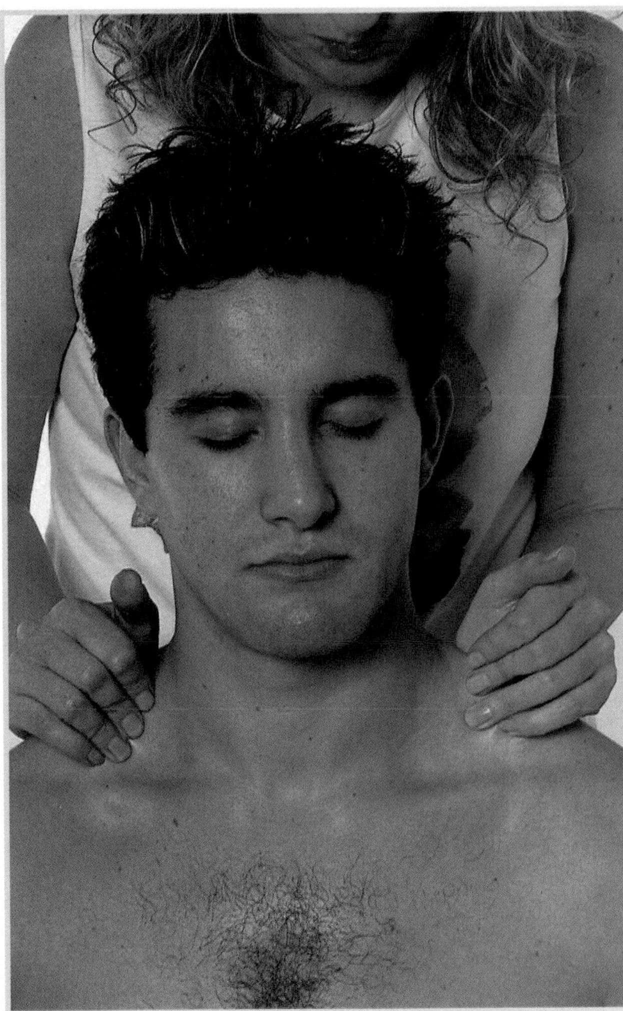

2 Press the heels of your hands into the back of your partner's shoulders and then gently roll the muscles forward, over the top of the shoulders. (This movement is particularly effective when working on someone who has broad shoulders.)

Practice 5

Wringing the shoulders

1 Place both of your hands on top of one of your partner's shoulders.

2 Pick up the muscle with one hand, then squeeze and pull it towards you. Repeat the procedure using the other hand. Working rhythmically all over the shoulder area, repeat this action, picking up as much muscle as you can while alternating hands.

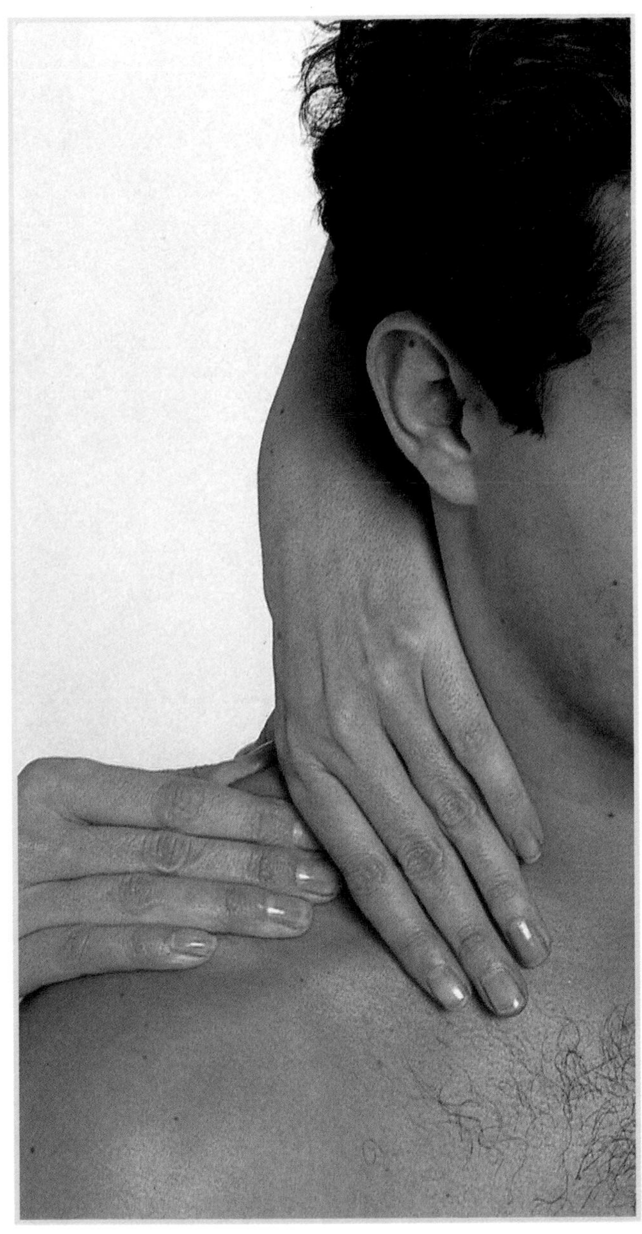

Repeat steps 1 and 2 on the receiver's other shoulder.

Friction

FRICTIONS ARE SMALL, circular movements that penetrate deeply into the tissues, causing the muscle to be moved against the bone (as when working near the spine) or the skin to be moved over the bone (as when moving the skin over the bones of the scalp).

Note that friction differs from rubbing, a much lighter technique whereby your hand moves over the surface of the skin, the heat in that area being increased by the friction. Rubbing usually involves the ball or heel of the hand. By contrast, the balls of the thumbs are usually employed when carrying out friction technique, although the pads of the fingers and the heels of the hands are also commonly used, and even the knuckles or elbows.

To perform friction, place your thumbs on the area to be worked on and move them using small, circular motions. Start off gently, and then use your body weight to increase the pressure. Try using your knuckles on particularly troublesome areas, too. Knotted muscles can be rather tender, but the receiver usually experiences great relief as the tension is released.

Note that although deep friction with the thumbs is suitable for the upper back and shoulders, it is unsuitable for the head because it exerts strong pressure.

THE BENEFITS OF FRICTION

Friction is beneficial because it:

- *breaks down knots and nodules of tension;*
- *increases the blood supply, thereby bringing fresh oxygen and nutrients;*
- *eliminates waste deposits;*
- *breaks down old scar tissue;*
- *relieves pain;*
- *breaks down fatty deposits;*
- *improves skin condition.*

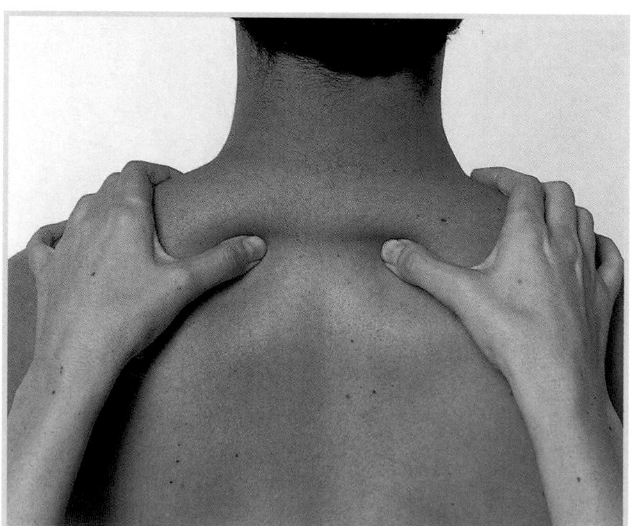

Practice 1

Frictioning the upper back

Stand behind the receiver and place the pads of your thumbs on the receiver's upper back, level with the base of the shoulder blades.

1 Lean into your thumbs as you perform small, deep, circular movements, working outwards up the back.

Caution

Do not press directly on to the spine.

2 If you find a 'knotty' area, either perform extra friction over the troublesome spot or press into it with your thumbs, maintaining the pressure for a few seconds before relaxing it.

3 You can continue the friction by working up the neck until you reach the base of the skull, but remember that you must always friction the neck gently.

Practice 2

Frictioning around the shoulder blades

Use your thumbs to friction around the shoulder blades. Alternatively, you could use the heel of your hand.

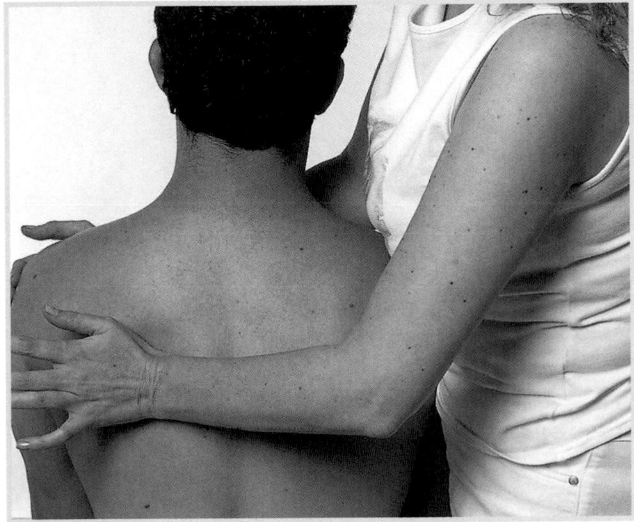

Place your right arm over the front of the receiver's right shoulder and the heel of your left hand against the lower medial (inside) edge of the scapula (shoulder blade). Using strong pressure and small movements, rotate the heel of your hand as you work up to the top of the shoulder blade.

Repeat step 1 on the receiver's right shoulder.

Practice 4

Rubbing under the skull

Remember that rubbing is different from friction. This technique involves rubbing your hand (usually the heel or the ball) gently and briskly over the surface of the skin.

Place one hand gently on the receiver's forehead to support their head. With your fingers pointing upwards, place the heel of your other hand against the base of the skull (occiput) and lightly rub over the surface of the skin.

Practice 3

Frictioning under the skull

This technique is excellent for preventing tension headaches.

Place one hand on the receiver's forehead for support. Position the fingertips of your other hand at the base of the skull (occiput). Gently make circular friction movements around the base of the skull.

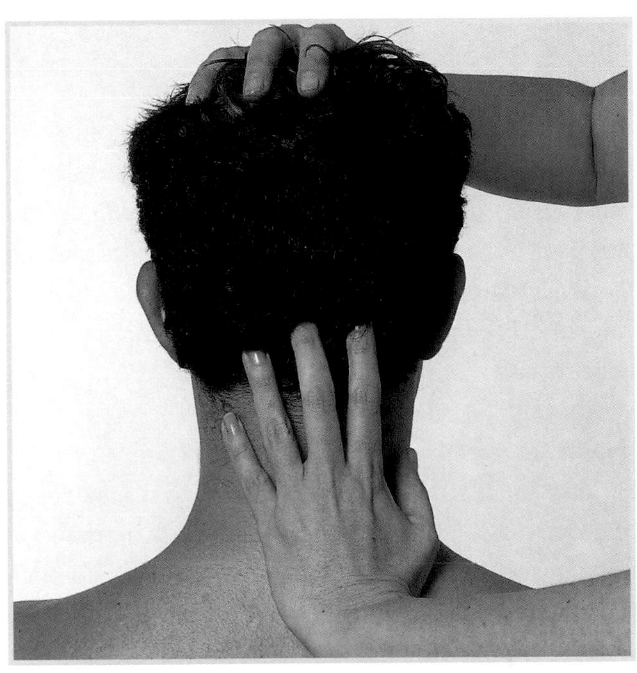

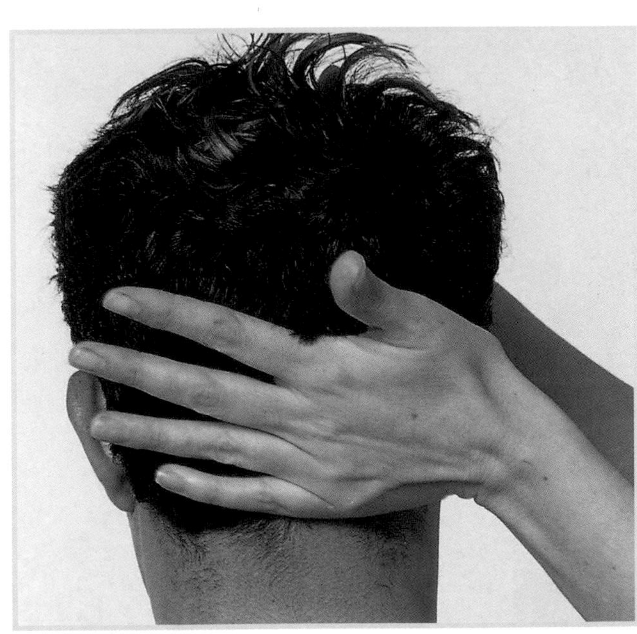

Tapotement

TAPOTEMENT MOVEMENTS are also known as percussion movements. In classical Swedish massage, tapotement includes cupping, hacking, flicking and even beating and pounding! Tapotement for Indian head massage, however, includes hacking, flicking, champi or champissage (double hacking), tapping (tabla playing) and cupping.

Tapotement movements should be light and springy, for which the wrists need to be loose and flexible.

Hacking

Hacking is performed with the outer edges of your hands. Keeping your wrists loose and flexible, hold your hands in front of you, thumbs uppermost, with the palms facing each other. Flick your hands up and down alternately in a brisk, rhythmical way. Make sure that the movements are coming from the wrist. (If you keep your elbows tucked in you will not be tempted to use your upper arms.)

Your hacking should be light and bouncy and should not resemble a heavy chopping action. Flicking is a lighter version of hacking and is sometimes referred to as 'finger-hacking'. The difference between hacking and flicking is that flicking involves the sides of the little fingers only, not the edge of the hands.

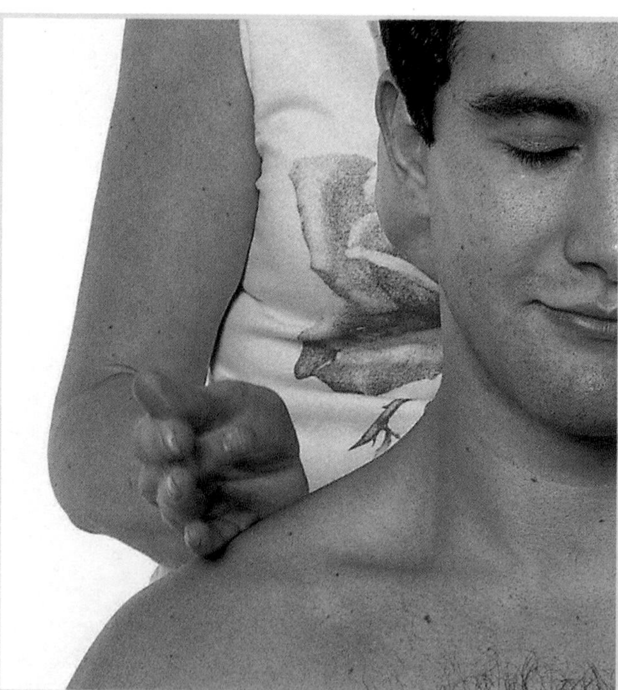

Champi (double hacking)

Champi is similar to hacking, the difference being that both hands are used at the same time (when hacking, your hands move one after the other).

Place your hands in a praying position and then relax them, allowing the heels of your hands and your fingertips to remain in gentle contact. Using your little fingers, now make light, rapid, striking movements on the area being treated.

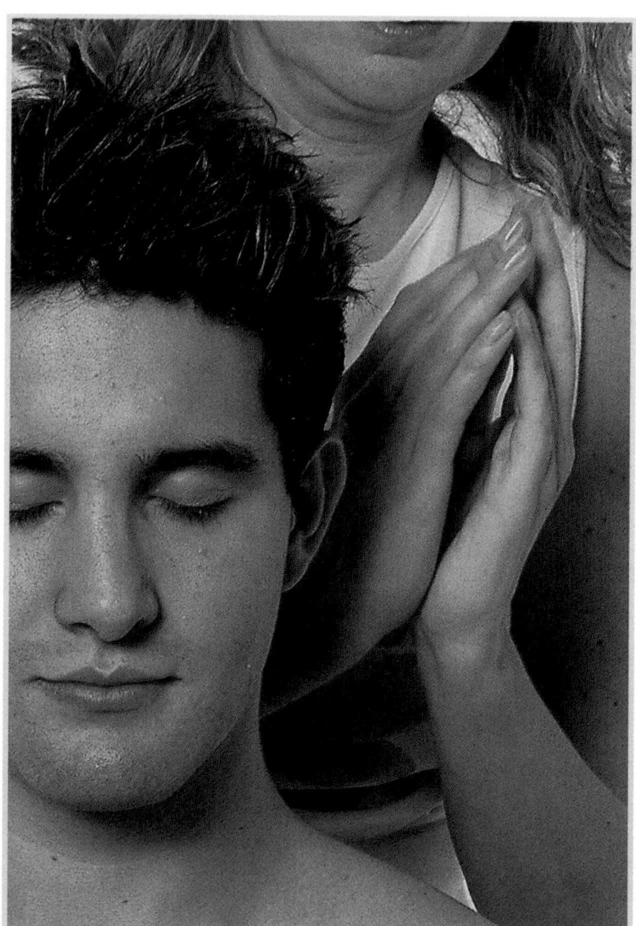

Tapping (tabla playing)

The word 'tabla' is probably derived from the Arabic word *tabl*, referring to the primary drum used in both the classical and popular music of northern India.

Tapping, or tabla playing, is a very light technique that can be used on all areas of the body; for example, while hacking and champi (double hacking) are not suitable for the top of the head or face, tapping is ideal.

Tapping is performed by gently tapping the fingertips on the area being treated. The technique may be performed using just one or two fingertips (for instance, the tips of the index and middle fingers), one finger followed by another or all of the fingers at once. The rhythm can be varied: slow tapping is soothing, whereas rapid tapping is energising and stimulating.

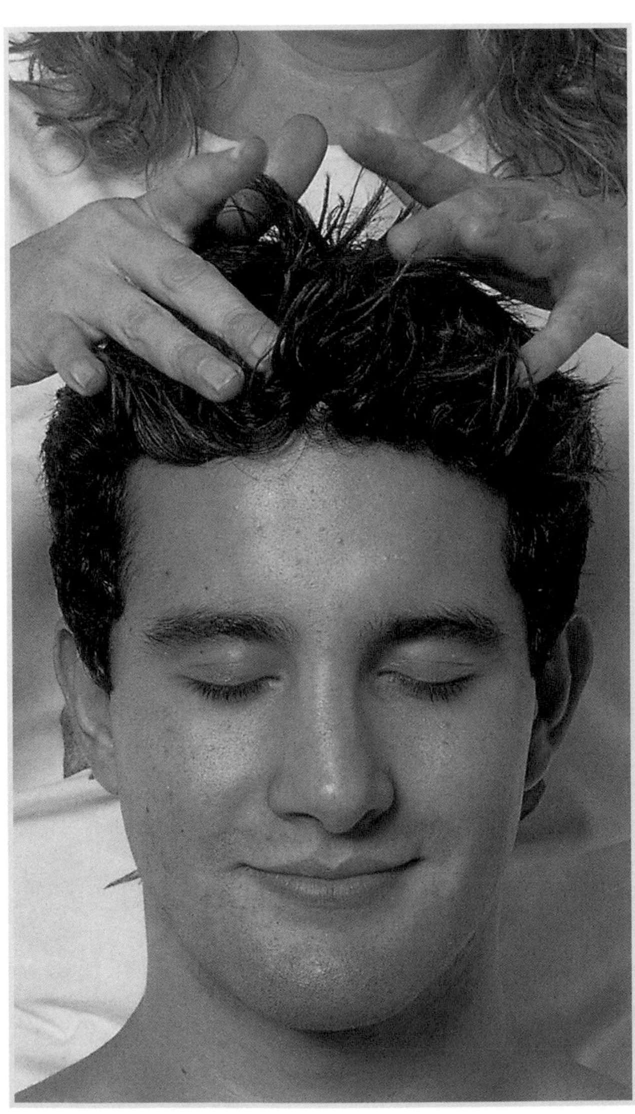

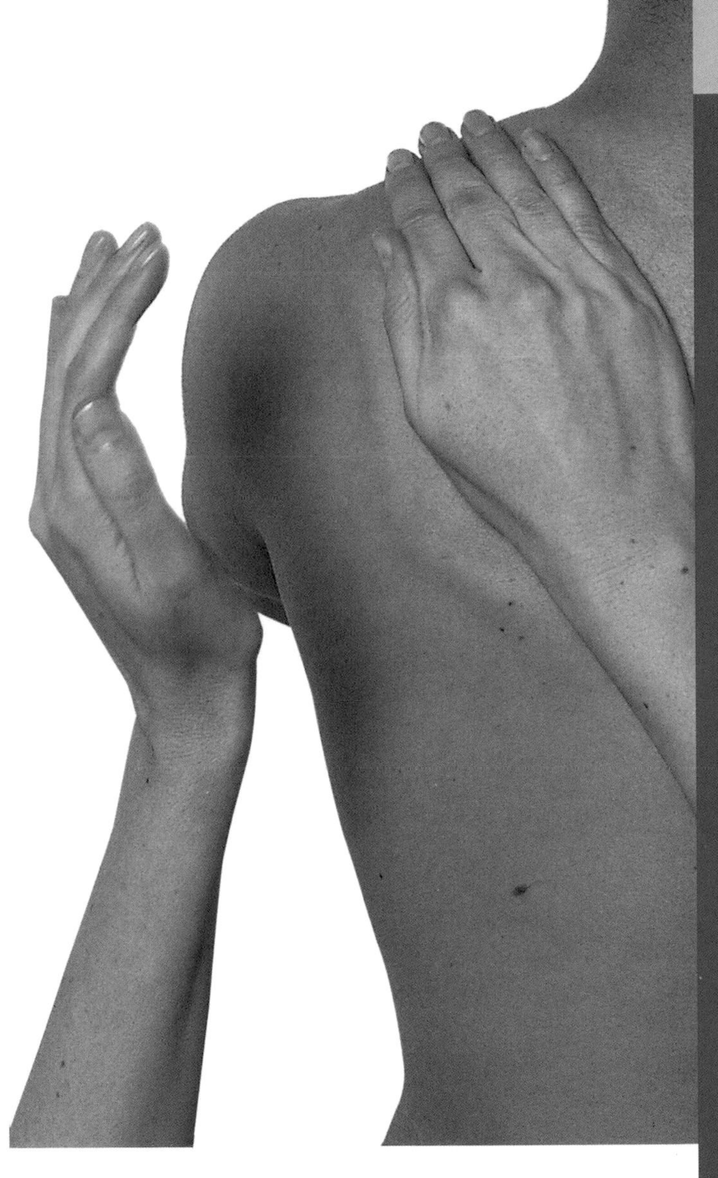

Cupping

To perform cupping, a hollow curve is first made with the fingers and thumbs of each hand, the cupped hands then being brought down on the body in quick succession. If this movement is performed correctly, a distinctly hollow sound, rather like a trotting horse, can be heard. A slapping noise should not, however, be produced.

THE BENEFITS OF TAPOTEMENT

Tapotement is beneficial because it:

- *stimulates and energises the mind;*
- *stimulates the circulation;*
- *improves muscle tone;*
- *reduces fatty deposits;*
- *loosens mucus in the lungs.*

Practice 1

Hacking across the shoulders

Position yourself behind the receiver and place your hands above the receiver's shoulders, with your palms facing each other and your thumbs uppermost.

1 Keeping your elbows tucked in, and with loose wrists, strike the top of the shoulders with the outer edges of your hands in a brisk and rhythmic way. Make sure that you are using a light and gentle action – no karate chopping!

2 For an even lighter effect (i.e., flicking), perform the same movement, but this time using the sides of your little fingers only.

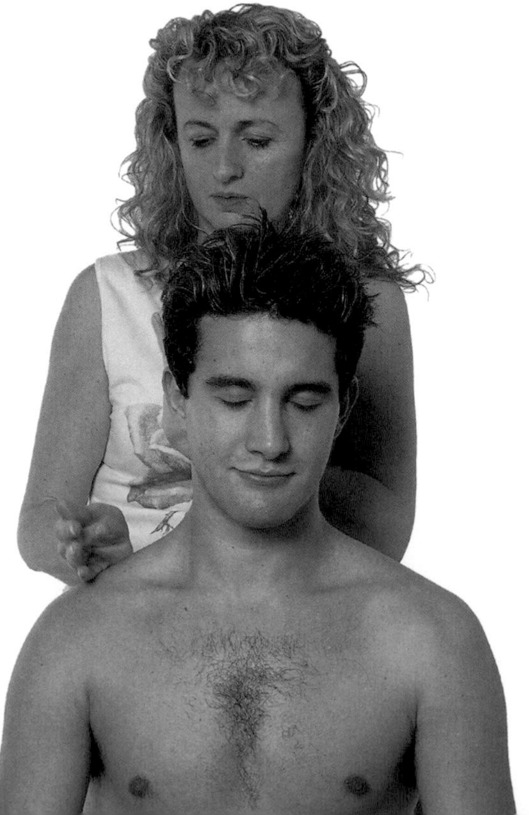

Practice 2

Champi or double hacking across the shoulders

Place your hands in the prayer position and then allow them to relax so that the heels of your hands and fingertips remain in gentle contact.

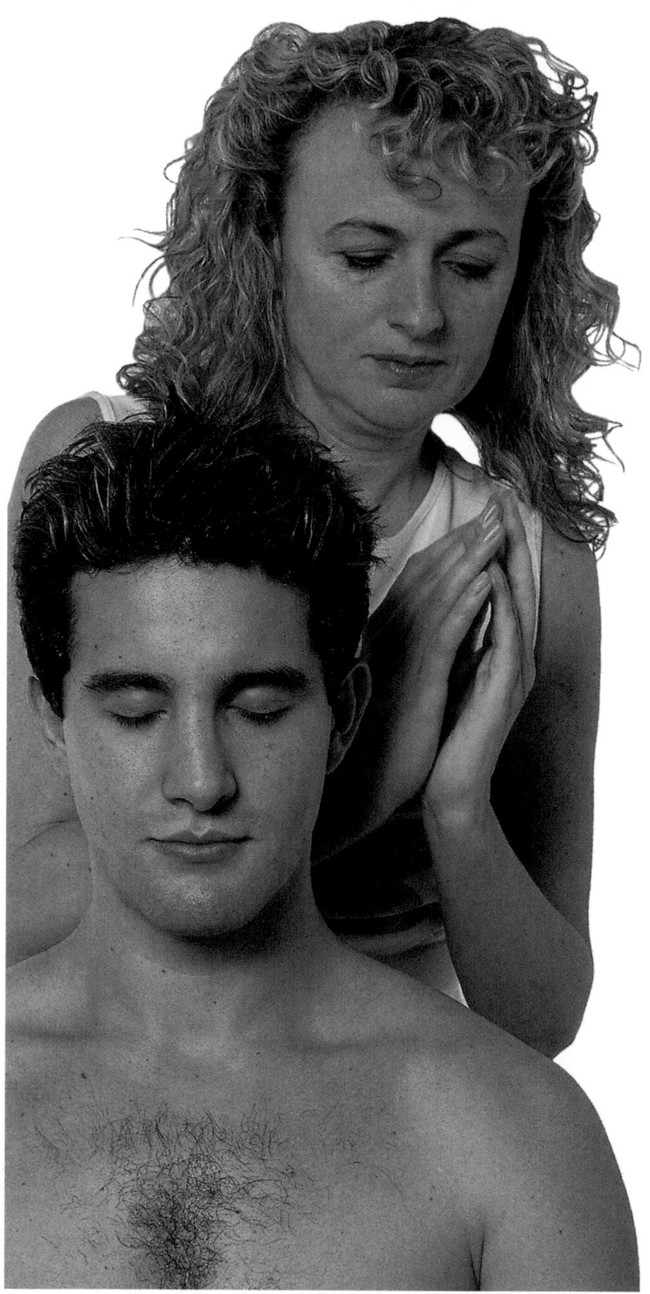

Make light, rapid, striking movements with your little fingers all across the receiver's shoulders. Your partner should feel stimulated and energised as a result.

Practice 3

Tapping or tabla playing on the scalp

Hold your hands above the receiver's scalp and then gently tap, or drum, your fingertips all over your partner's head.

As you bounce your fingertips off the receiver's hair in quick, light movements, it should feel as though raindrops are falling gently on the ground. Try drumming on the receiver's scalp using only two fingertips (either those of your index and middle fingers or of your middle and fourth fingers). Now tap using all of your fingertips at once and notice how different this method feels.

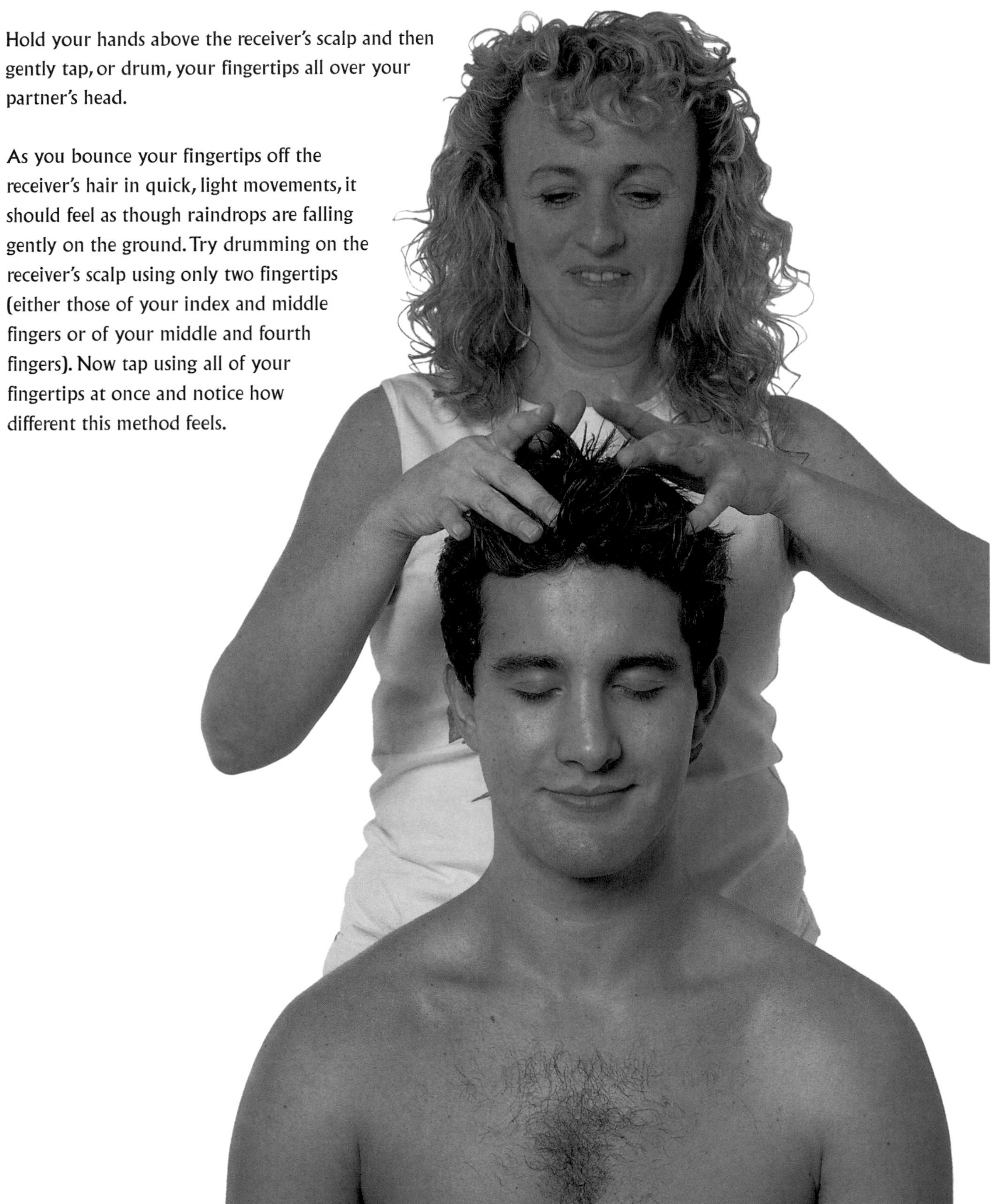

Practice 4

Cupping the upper back

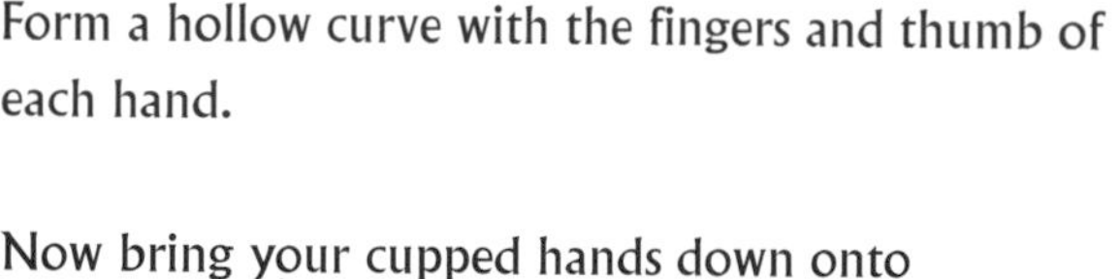

Form a hollow curve with the fingers and thumb of each hand.

Now bring your cupped hands down onto the receiver's upper back in rapid succession. Listen for the hollow sound that should be produced as your cupped hands create a vacuum. (Note that although reddening, or erythema, of the skin will quickly result as blood is brought to the surface, cupping should not be uncomfortable for the receiver.)

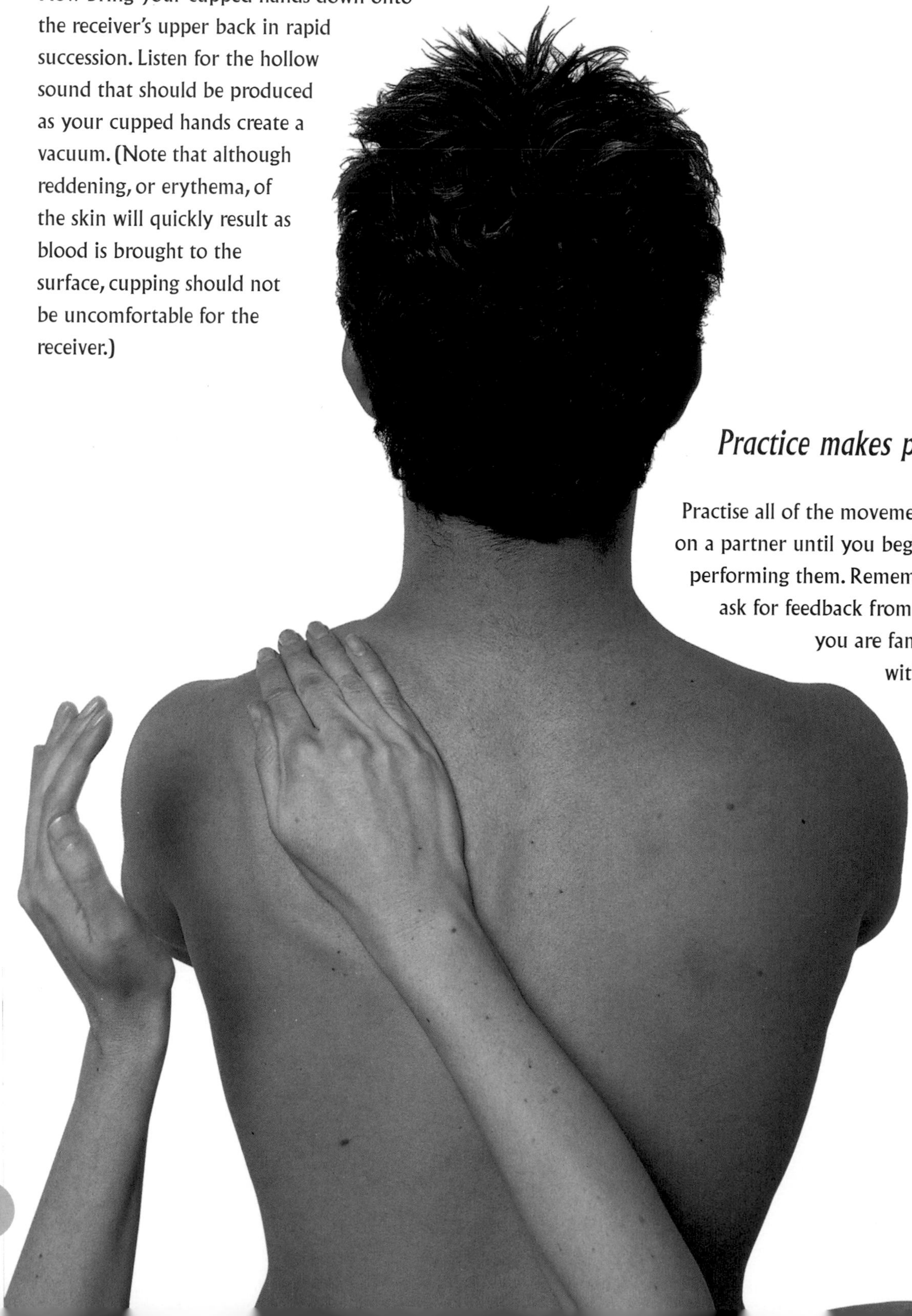

Practice makes perfect

Practise all of the movements in this chapter on a partner until you begin to feel confident performing them. Remember, too, always to ask for feedback from your partner while you are familiarising yourself with the techniques. Once you have mastered these movements, start to follow your intuition and allow your own, unique movements to develop.

The Chakras and Indian Head Massage

AN INDIAN HEAD MASSAGE is not complete until the chakras, which are described in earliest-recorded Indian history, are balanced. The ancient Sanskrit word chakra means 'wheel', 'circle' or 'disc' and chakras are thought to be spinning vortices of energy. Non-physical energy centres located a few centimetres away from the physical body, chakras act as a bridge that links the physical with the energies of the subtle body. If the chakras are blocked, disease can manifest itself, but when the chakras are freed from negative energies and blockages, balance and health is restored. Aligning the chakras will therefore increase the physical, mental, emotional and subtle benefits of an Indian head massage.

Although many therapists concentrate on the three higher chakras only, in my opinion all of the energy centres need to be worked on to restore the balance of inner peace and harmony. If the lower chakras are not given equal emphasis, the receiver will feel disconnected and ungrounded.

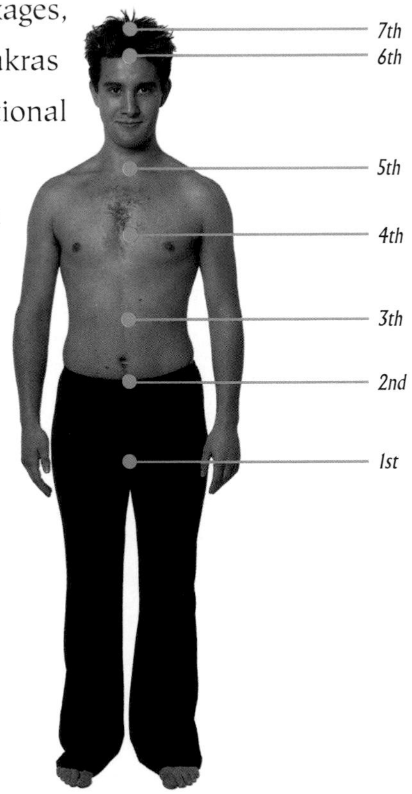

The lower chakras

THERE ARE THOUGHT TO BE SEVEN MAJOR CHAKRAS, AS FOLLOWS.

1 *The base chakra, Muladhara.*
2 *The sacral chakra, Svadhisthana.*
3 *The solar plexus chakra, Manipura.*
4 *The heart chakra, Anahata.*
5 *The throat chakra, Visuddha.*
6 *The brow chakra, Ajna.*
7 *The crown chakra, Sahasrara.*

The base chakra
(also known as the root or earth chakra)

Sanskrit name: Muladhara.
Location: Between the anus and the genitals.
Colour: Red.
Element: Earth.
Associated glands: The adrenals (some say the testes or ovaries).
Sound: 'Lam'.
Function: The base chakra is our connection with the physical world. It is associated with stability, security and our survival. Also known as the earth or root chakra, it provides us with the solid ground upon which we can build our lives. It enables us to perceive the earth as a safe, secure place that satisfies all of our needs.
Imbalance: If the base chakra is not functioning correctly, you may be lacking in stamina. Feelings of uncertainty and worry will surround you. You may have the sensation that you are floating, as though you are not connected to the earth.
Physical problems: Problems relating to the spine, bones, teeth, nails, ankles and knees may be experienced if the base chakra is imbalanced. Digestive disorders, particularly of the rectum, anus and colon, are also common.

The sacral chakra
(also known as the sexual or abdomen chakra)

Sanskrit name: Svadhisthana.
Location: Lower abdomen, above the genitals.
Colour: Orange.
Element: Water.
Associated glands: The testes or ovaries (some say the spleen).
Sound: 'Vam'.
Function: The sacral chakra is concerned with sexuality, reproduction, pleasure and desire. Its element, water, continually produces new life, and so it is through the sacral chakra that we also create new life. The water element purifies, too, and

dissolves away blockages, enabling our feelings to flow freely.

Imbalance: If the sacral chakra is disharmonious, there will be problems with the sexual organs and in forming sexual relationships. An imbalanced sex drive can lead to frigidity and, if the sex drive is shut off, impotence. Alternatively, there may be excessive sexual impulses resulting in promiscuity or, in some cases, sexual perversion.

Physical problems: The sexual chakra often becomes disharmonious during puberty, a time when the sexual energies awaken, and many parents are unfortunately incapable of teaching their children how to use them. Because this chakra is connected with the water element, problems may also arise with the kidneys and bladder.

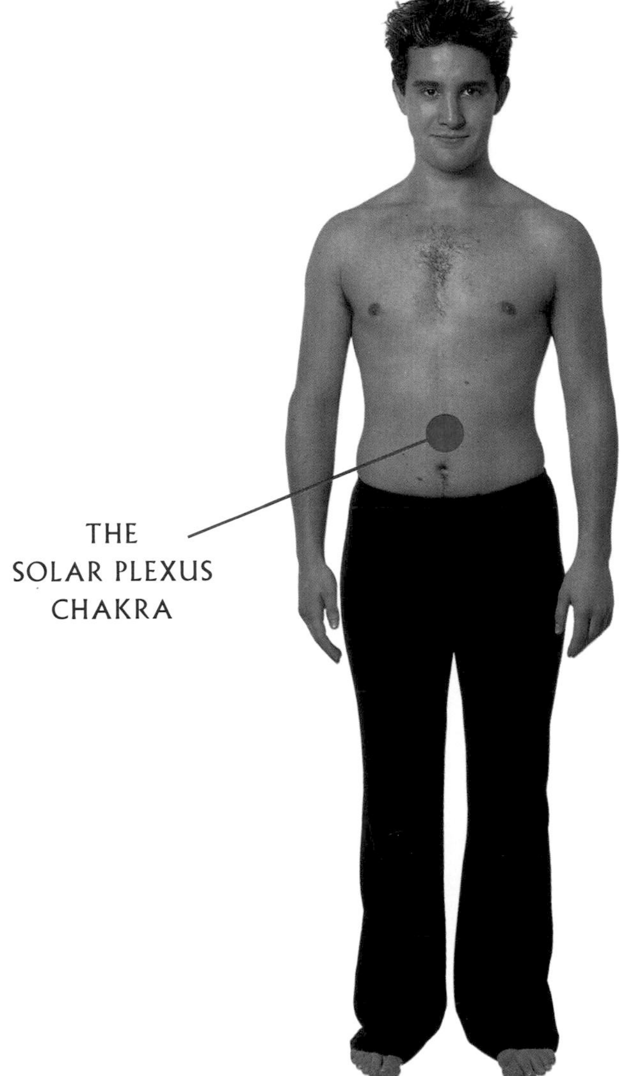

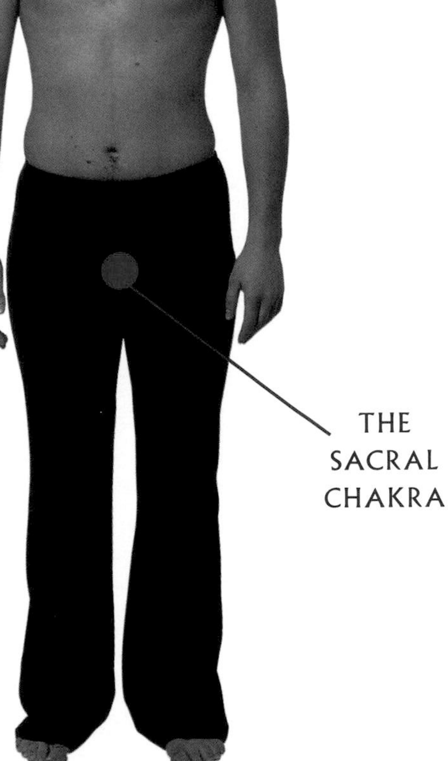

The solar plexus chakra

(also known as the navel or power chakra)

Sanskrit name:	Manipura.
Location:	Just above the navel.
Colour:	Yellow.
Element:	Fire.
Associated glands:	The pancreas (some say the adrenals).
Sound:	'Ram'.
Function:	The solar plexus chakra is our sun, our centre of power. If this chakra is balanced, we feel full of joy and energy, yet also at peace and in harmony with ourselves. It is from this chakra that we transform our desires and emotions into action.

	The solar plexus chakra is also concerned with transforming our food into energy and with separating the useful from the not so useful.
Imbalance:	If the solar plexus chakra is disharmonious, there will be an inner restlessness and lack of contentment. This agitation and inability to relax is often coupled with a lack of self-esteem and self-confidence.
Physical problems:	The physical problems that may be manifested by a disharmonious solar plexus chakra include digestive problems, such as diabetes and ulcers, and eating disorders like anorexia, allergies and chronic fatigue.

The heart chakra

Sanskrit name:	Anahata.
Location:	The centre of the chest.
Colour:	Green or pink.
Element:	Air.
Associated gland:	The thymus.
Sound:	'Yam'.
Function:	The heart chakra is the centre of the chakra system, a bridge that connects the three lower, physical and emotional centres to the three higher, mental and spiritual centres. The fourth chakra is connected with unconditional love, compassion and empathy. If the heart chakra is open, then the higher abilities of the brow, or third-eye, chakra will develop at the same time (many spiritual schools, in both the East and the West, therefore focus on opening the heart chakra).
Imbalance:	Malfunction of this chakra can lead to sadness, depression and a fear of rejection. There may also be an inability to give and receive love.
Physical problems:	The physical problems that may be manifested if this chakra is imbalanced include blood-pressure, heart and circulatory problems, as well as disorders of the lungs.

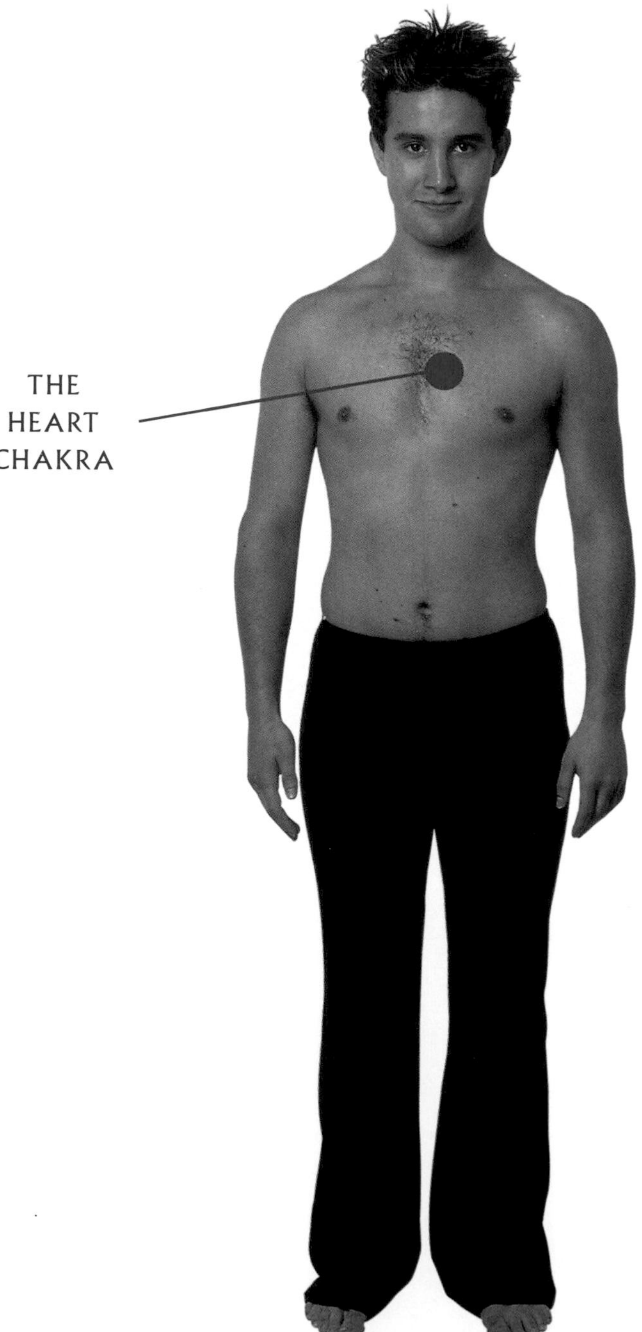

The higher chakras

The throat chakra

Sanskrit name: Visuddha.
Location: The throat.
Colour: Blue.
Element: Sound or ether.
Associated gland: The thyroid.
Sound: 'Ham'.

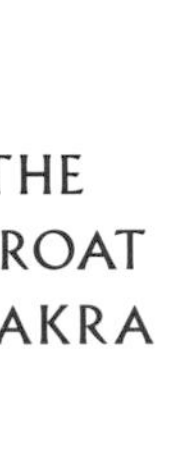

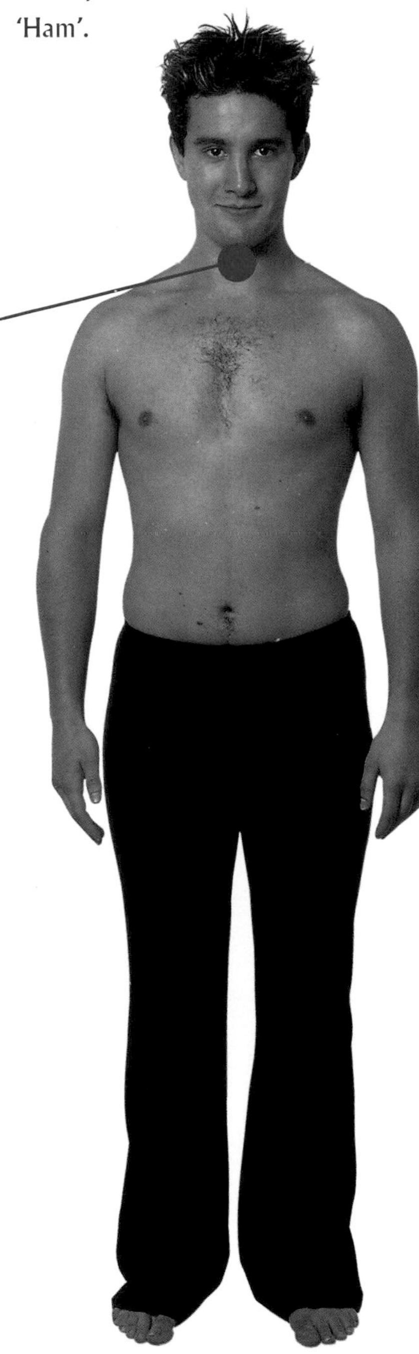

Function: The throat chakra is connected with communication and self-expression. It is also concerned with speaking one's truth and the true expression of the soul without fearing what others think. From this centre, we listen to our inner voice. Through it, we express the contents of all of the other chakras to the world.

Imbalance: Psychological imbalances associated with this chakra include an inability to express one's emotions.

Physical problems: The physical problems arising from an imbalance of the throat chakra include all ear, nose and throat disorders, as well as any disorders of the voice, such as stuttering. Physical problems with the neck, shoulders and jaw, as well as thyroid disorders, may also arise.

The brow chakra
(also known as the third-eye chakra)

Sanskrit name: Ajna.
Location: The centre of the forehead.
Colour: Indigo.
Element: Light.
Associated glands: The pituitary (some say the pineal).
Sound: 'Om'.
Function: The brow chakra is associated with intuition and inner vision and wisdom. It enables us to perceive the world in a new way and to become aware of other dimensions of reality.

Imbalance: If this chakra is out of balance, it can lead to a lack of intuition and a total disbelief in anything that cannot be proven scientifically.
If the 'third eye', as the brow chakra is also known, is open and the base chakra in particular is not grounding you properly, you may become very confused, hallucinate and lose touch with reality (this is why all of the chakras should be balanced and not just the higher chakras).

Physical problems: The problems that can result from an imbalance of the brow chakra include visual disorders, nightmares and headaches.

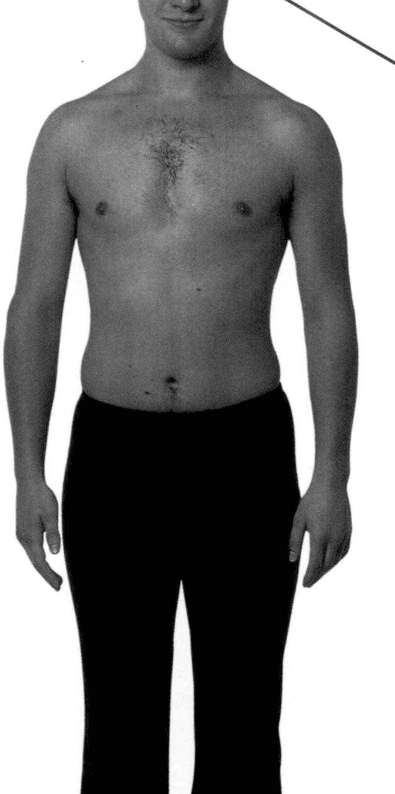

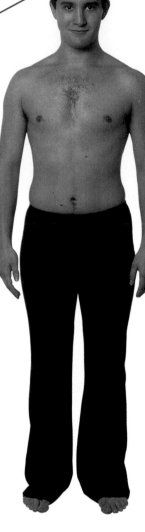

THE
CROWN
CHAKRA

The crown chakra

Sanskrit name: Sahasrara.

Location: The top of the head.

Colour: Violet.

Element: Thought or knowing.

Associated glands: The pineal (some say the pituitary).

Sound: A silent 'om' or silence.

Function: The crown chakra is concerned with understanding, bliss and enlightenment. It is our link with the divine, enabling us to become at one with our creator.

Imbalance: Disturbances in the crown chakra can cause an unwillingness to, and fear of, opening up one's spiritual potential. Alienation and confusion may be present.

Physical problems: The problems associated with an imbalance of the crown chakra include epilepsy, Alzheimer's disease and Parkinson's disease.

Balancing the chakras

THE CHAKRAS ARE BALANCED at the end of an Indian head massage to impart a sense of inner peace and harmony. By the end of the treatment, the person on whom you are working will be deeply relaxed and will therefore be much more receptive to subtle techniques.

As I have already stated, I feel that it is vital to pay attention to all of the chakras, and not just to the higher energy centres. Working on the higher chakras alone can result in the receiver feeling very light-headed or spaced out and extremely ungrounded or disconnected with the earth. Some individuals may even feel dizzy and out of touch with reality.

Step–by–step chakra balancing

Before starting, make sure that you and your partner will not be disturbed. Remember to create the right ambience, as described on pages 18 to 19 before commencing the chakra balancing treatment.

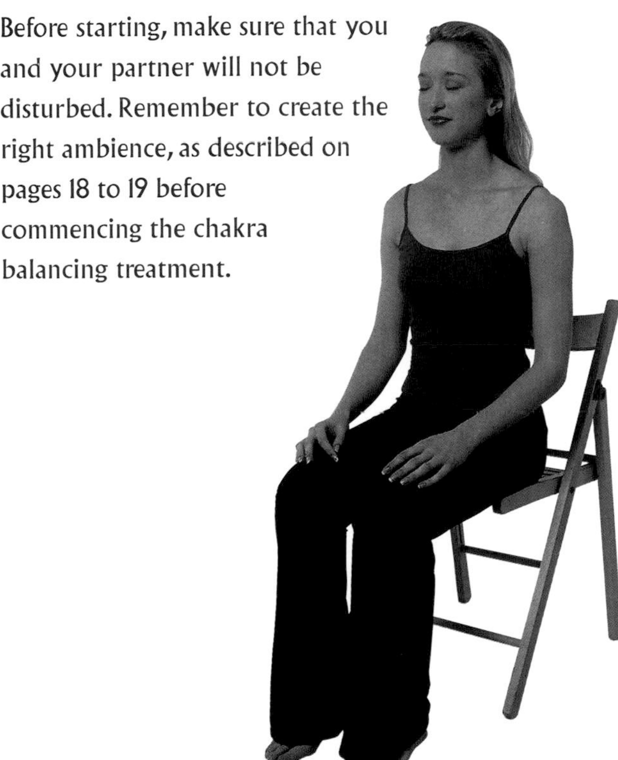

1 Ensure that your partner is sitting comfortably, with his or her back straight and feet placed flat on the floor. Because crossed legs will impair the flow of energy, also make sure that their legs are uncrossed.

2 Stand behind the receiver with your arms hanging loosely by your sides. It's important that you feel grounded, so visualise roots extending from your feet deep into the earth, thereby establishing a secure connection.

3 To establish an energy connection, gently place your hands on your partner's shoulders. Close your eyes and visualise a healing light descending from above and surrounding you and your partner.

4 Take a few deep breaths and then allow your breathing to become synchronised with that of your partner. Feel any stress dissolving away and imagine it being released through both of your 'roots', all the way down into the centre of the earth.

5 Gently remove your hands from your partner's shoulders. Now position yourself at the receiver's side. Let your hands hover a few centimetres above his or her head and try to tune into the energy of the chakras. Take note of any sensations that you may feel, such as a feeling of heat or tingling.

6 Without touching the receiver's physical body, slowly move your hands down the chakras, one palm scanning the front of the body while the other palm scans the back.

7 As you reach the base of the spine, allow your hands to hover a few centimetres away from the receiver's body and try to sense the base chakra. Vary the distance of your hands from the receiver's body to discover your most receptive position. Visualise a clear, deep-red colour emanating from this chakra.

Now move your hands up a little to the sacral chakra, which is positioned slightly below the navel. Sense the circular motion of the sacral chakra and visualise a clear, orange colour radiating from this energy centre.

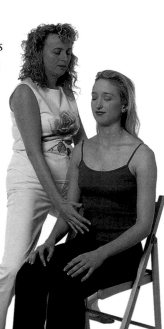

Let your hands rise to the solar plexus chakra and feel it fill with a radiant golden light that glows brightly and clearly.

Allow your hands to wander up to the heart chakra, which is located in the centre of the chest. Sense a pink flower of light enfolded in its leaves of green, gently awakening and filling with the love vibration.

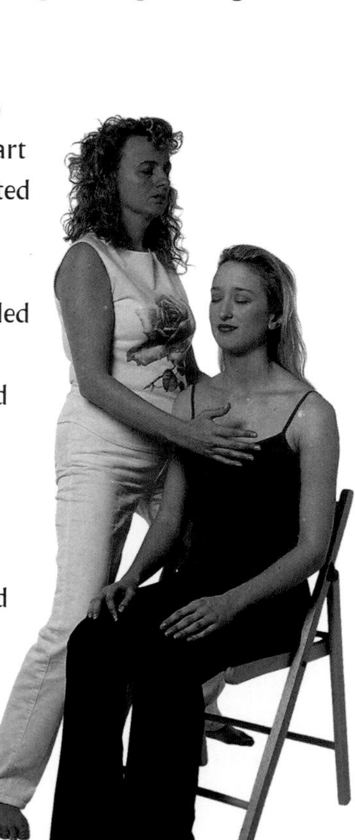

Move your hands to the throat chakra and visualise it filling and expanding with a radiant blue light.

Raise your hands to the brow chakra, from which you should visualise a beautiful indigo-blue light emerging.

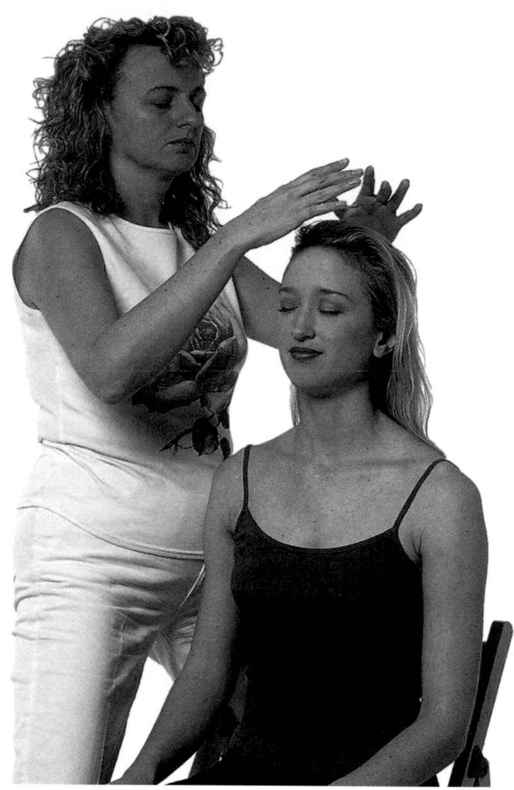

Finally, allow your hands to hover over the top of the receiver's head to sense the crown chakra. Visualise a bright, clear, violet light filling this centre.

Let your partner bathe in the waves of peace and harmony being produced and to experience the healing effects of the chakra balancing treatment.

8 Move in front of your partner and place your hands on their feet. Rub them gently to bring the receiver's consciousness back into their body and to ground them.

If you wish, you could give the receiver a grounding stone, such as smoky quartz, haematite, obsidian or black tourmaline, to hold. Ask your partner to open their eyes when they are ready.

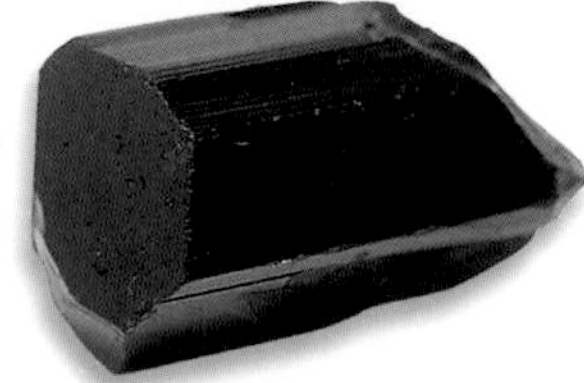

Step-by-Step Indian Head Massage

THE STEP-BY-STEP procedures in this chapter will enable you to carry out a complete Indian head massage on your friends and family.

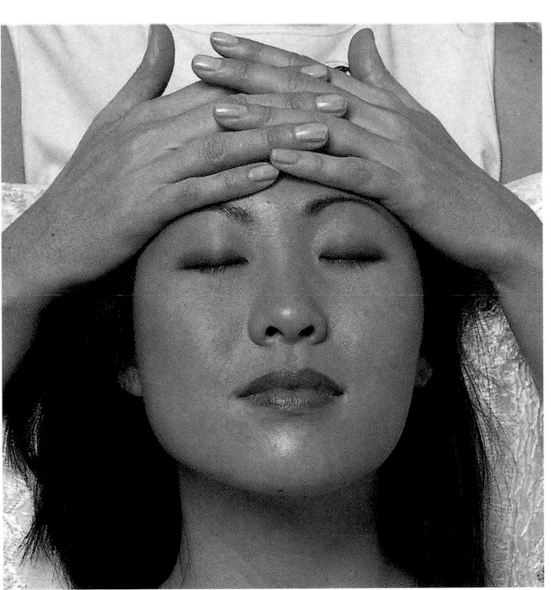

BEFORE YOU BEGIN

- *Make sure that you will be undisturbed for at least half an hour.*
- *Create a warm, relaxing, soothing environment (see pages 18 to 19).*
- *Ensure that everything that you will need – towels, pillows and oils (optional) – are close at hand.*
- *Wear comfortable, loose–fitting clothes.*
- *Make sure that your nails have been trimmed, wash your hands and remove any jewellery.*
- *Ask your partner to remove any earrings, necklaces, body–piercing jewellery or spectacles.*
- *Brush through your partner's hair.*
- *If your partner's hair is long, tie it up with a clip or other type of hair accessory to enable you to perform the upper back and neck massage.*
- *Check for any contraindications (see pages 23 to 24).*

MASSAGE TIPS

- *Be aware of your posture throughout the massage or you may need treatment afterwards!*
- *Maintain continuity of contact with the receiver throughout the massage. Once you have made a connection with your partner, try not to break it lest the flow of the massage is spoiled. One movement should flow into the next during an Indian head massage.*
- *Keep conversation to a minimum. Talking makes it difficult for you to concentrate and disturbs the flow of the treatment.*
- *Check that the receiver is comfortable. Ask them to let you know if there are any particular movements that they especially enjoy. You also need to know if they are experiencing any discomfort when you are working on a particular area.*
- *Experiment with using different pressures. Most people prefer a firm massage, particularly on the shoulders, but everyone is different. Start with fairly gentle stokes and gradually increase the pressure. Take care not to apply too much pressure to the face or any sensitive areas, however.*
- *Try using different rhythms. A slow rhythm will calm and soothe, whereas a brisk rhythm will energise and invigorate.*
- *Adapt your massage to partner's body language. Look out for any signs of discomfort during the treatment, such as tensing or flinching, as well as for signs of enjoyment, such as sighing, breathing deeply and other obvious signs of relaxation.*

Sequence A: the sitting position

ALLOW THIRTY MINUTES for this massage treatment. Indian head massage is traditionally given with the receiver seated. Make sure that receiver is sitting comfortably on a chair, that their legs are uncrossed and that their feet (ask them to remove their shoes) are placed flat on the ground. Place a pillow or cushion on the receiver's lap for them to rest their hands on. If they wish, you could place a crystal in each of their hands. Stand squarely behind your partner.

The upper back and shoulders sequence

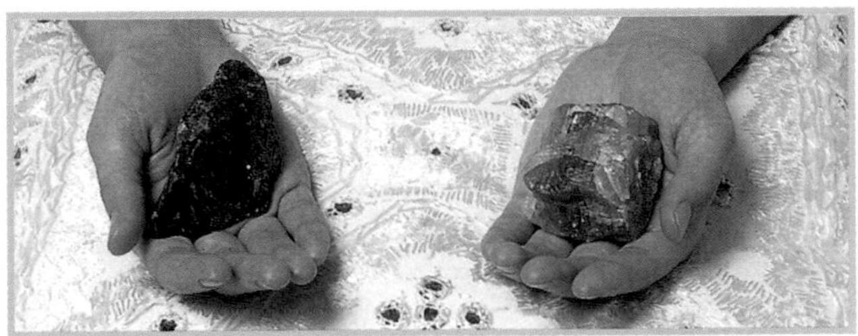

1 MAKING THE CONNECTION

Place your hands gently on the receiver's shoulders. First ask them to take a few deep breaths. Then ask them to breathe in peace and harmony and to breathe out any stress and tension.

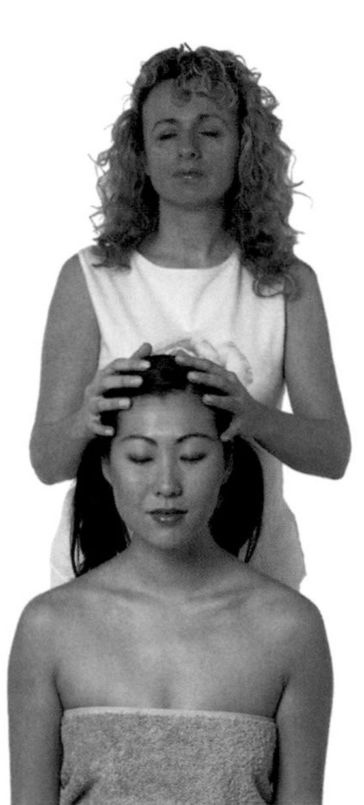

Now rest your hands very lightly on the receiver's head and leave them there for a minute or so until your partner feels completely relaxed.

> ***Caution***
> *Do not press down on the head. This would make the head, as well as the neck, feel uncomfortable.*

2 EFFLEURAGING THE UPPER BACK

Position yourself behind the receiver. Relax your hands and place a hand on either side of the spine on the receiver's upper back, level with the bottom of the shoulder blades, with your fingers facing upwards.

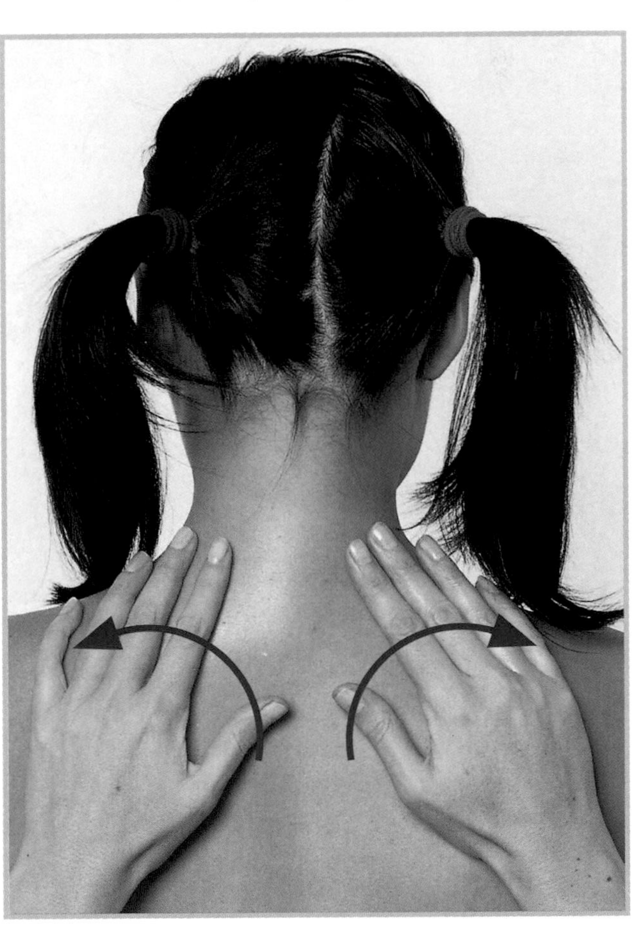

Using both hands simultaneously, perform large, stoking movements, working in an outward, circular direction. Work across the upper back and shoulders at least seven times.

3 FRICTIONING THE BACK

Stand or kneel behind the receiver and place the pads of your thumbs on the receiver's upper back, level with the base of the shoulder blades and a few centimetres away from the spine.

i) Using firm pressure, perform small, deep, circular movements with your thumbs as you gradually work your way up the back.

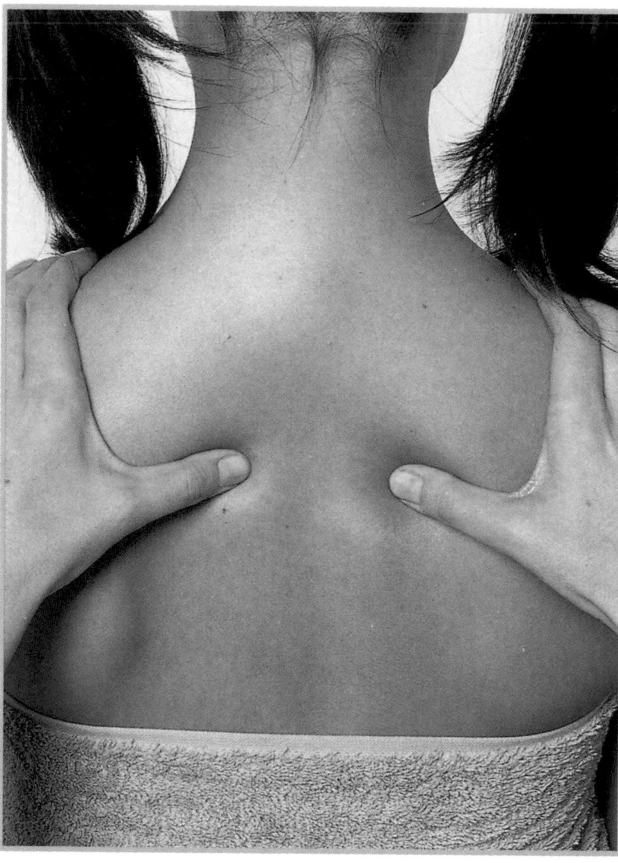

Caution

Do not press directly on the spine.

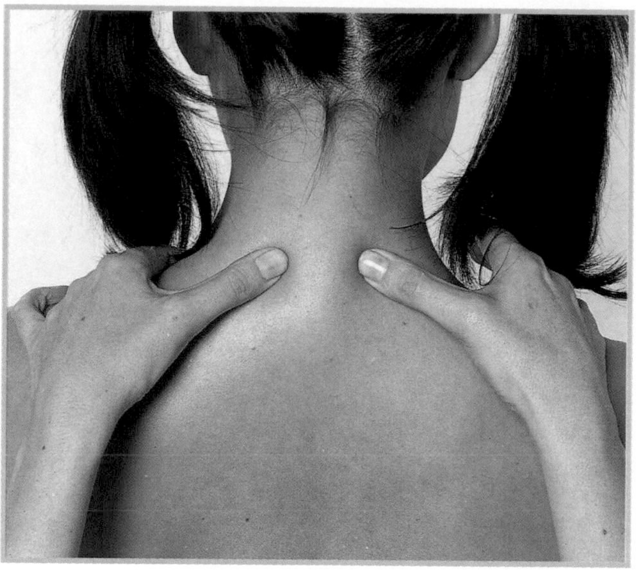

ii) When you reach the base of the neck, use more gentle pressure as you continue your friction up the neck.

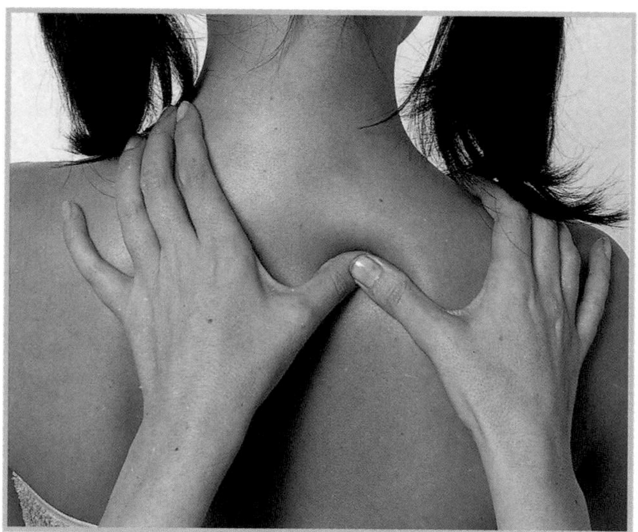

iii) Repeat the friction described in steps I and 2 very slowly, and if you encounter any knots and nodules of tension, spend extra time performing circular friction on these troublesome areas. Alternatively, place your thumbs (or one thumb on top of the other) on the area requiring attention and then press into it, if necessary using your body weight to exert firmer pressure. Maintain the pressure for a few seconds and then gradually release it. Repeat this movement until the discomfort in the area subsides.

4 PRESSING AND RELEASING THE BACK

Stand behind the receiver. Place the pads of your thumbs on the receiver's upper back, level with the base of the shoulder blades and a few centimetres away from the spine.

Using both thumbs simultaneously, press and release. Then move your thumbs slightly up the back and press and release again. Working up the back, continue this movement until you reach the neck.

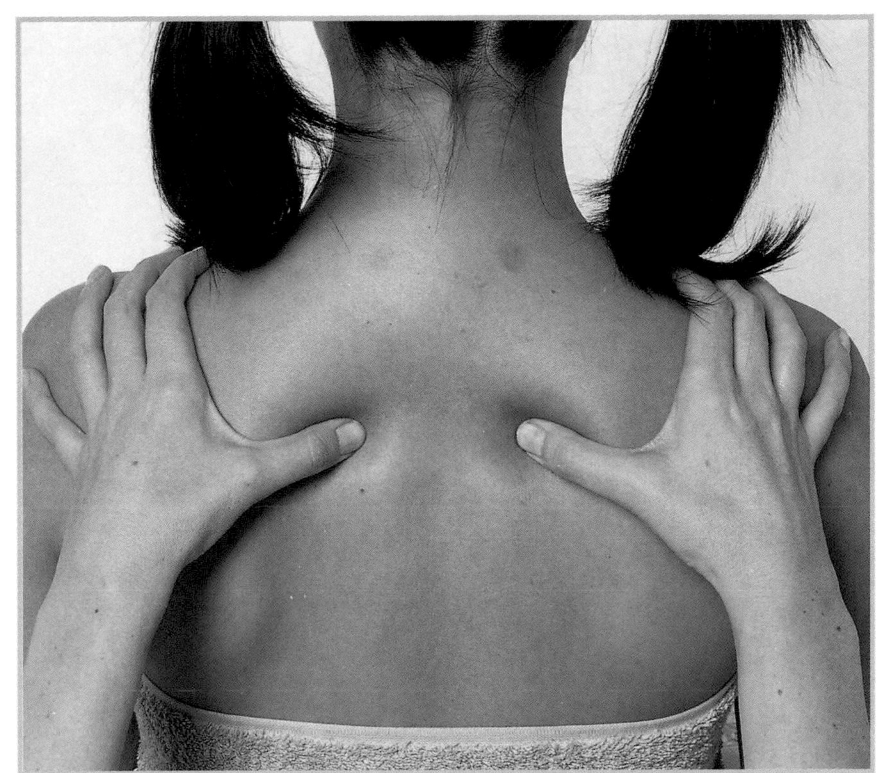

5 KNUCKLING THE BACK

Form your hands into fists and place them on the receiver's upper back, level with the base of the shoulder blades.

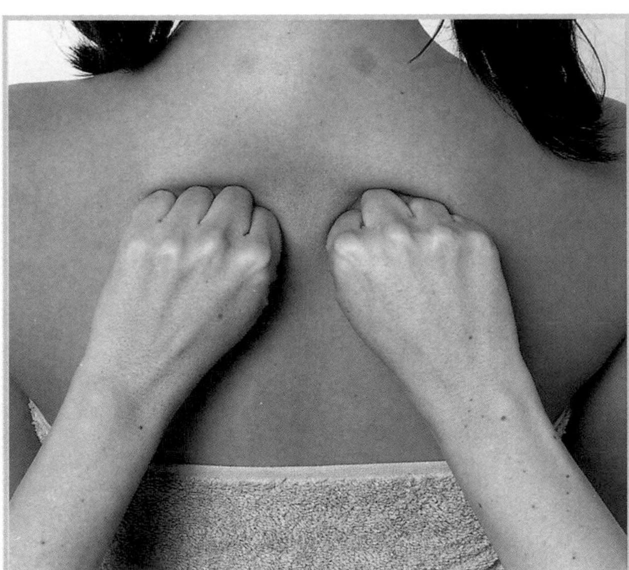

Use both hands simultaneously to knuckle up the whole of the upper back.

6 EFFLEURAGING THE LEFT SHOULDER BLADE

Stand to the side of the receiver. Place your right arm over the front of the receiver's shoulders and place your left hand on the left shoulder blade (scapula).

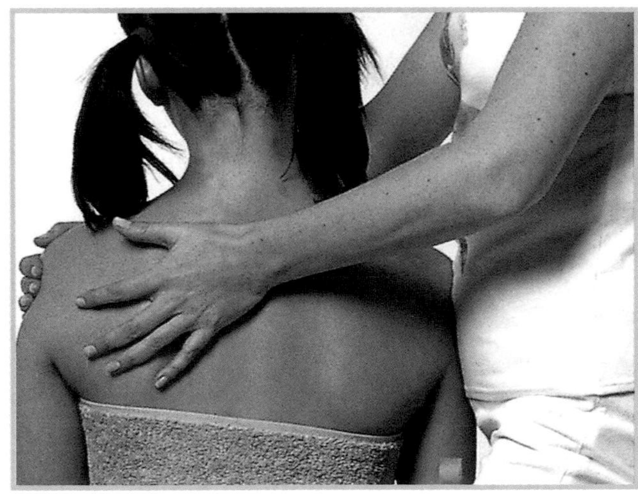

Use the palmar surface of your hand to circle around the shoulder blade. Repeat the procedure at least seven times.

7 RUBBING THE LEFT SHOULDER BLADE

Position yourself at the receiver's right side. Rest your right hand gently on the receiver's right shoulder and place the whole of your left hand on the left shoulder blade (scapula).

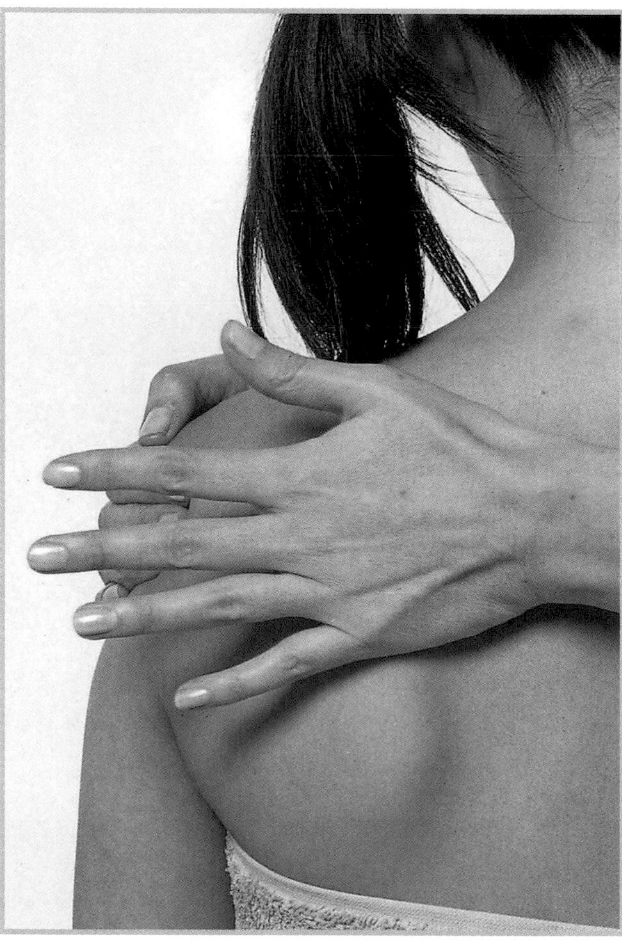

Use the whole of your hand to rub lightly and briskly across the top of the shoulder blade, between and below it. Continue rubbing until the area feels warm.

8 FRICTIONING THE LEFT SHOULDER BLADE

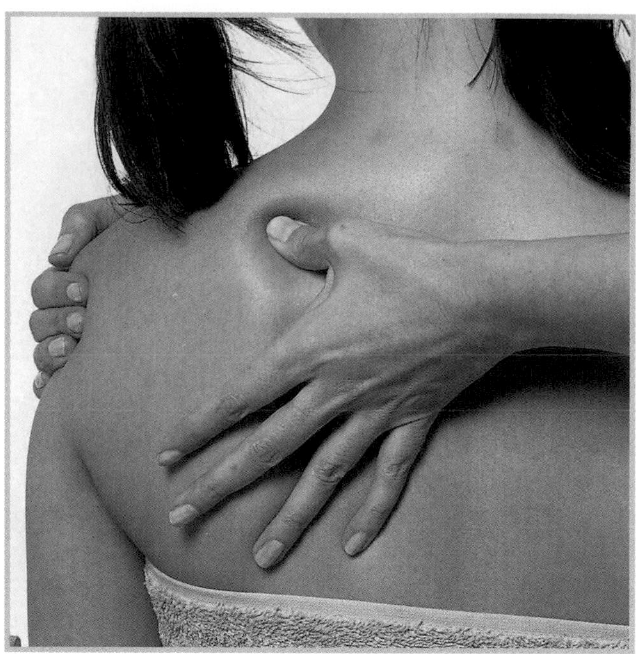

i) Standing to the side of the receiver, place your right arm over the front of your partner's left shoulder and position the thumb of your left hand at the bottom of the shoulder blade (scapula). Perform deep, circular, friction movements all around the shoulder blade, paying extra attention to any knots and nodules of tension.

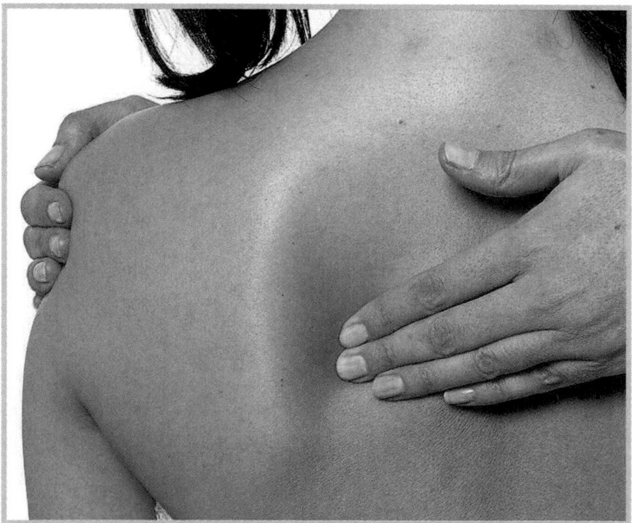

ii) Now try the same friction technique using your fingers instead of your thumb.

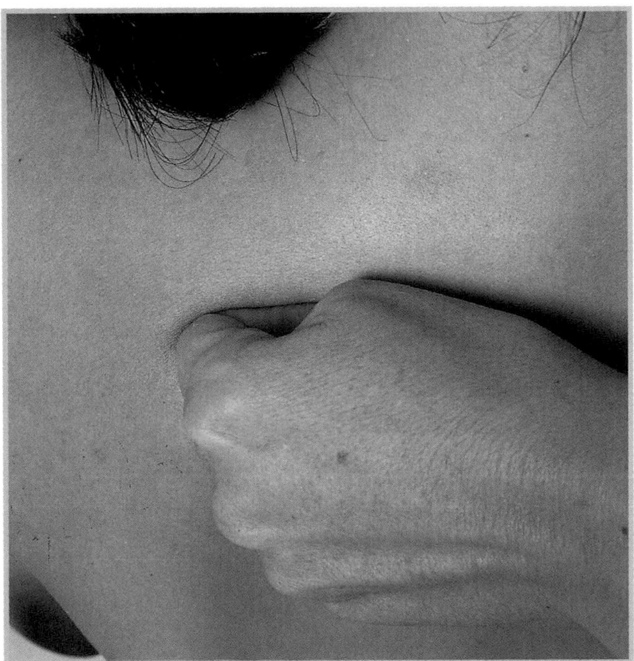

iii) Repeat the friction with your knuckles. This will allow you to penetrate deep into the tissues.

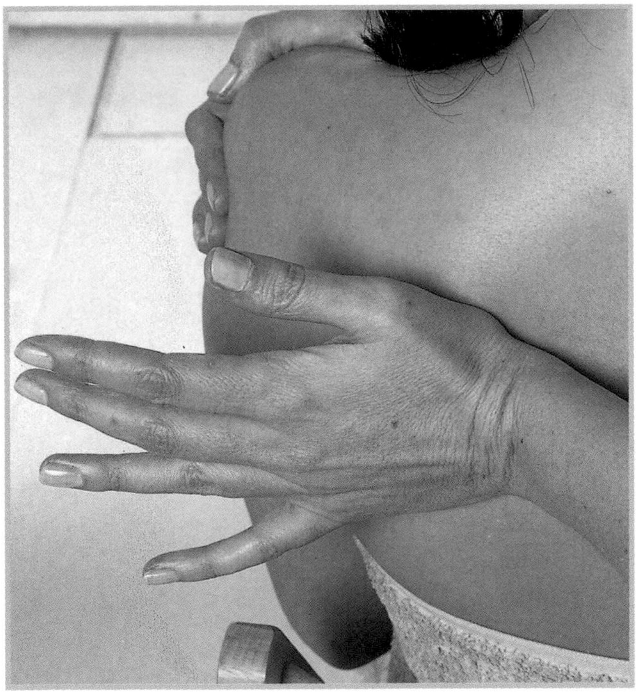

iv) Repeat this friction technique using the heel of your left hand, which should be placed against the inside edge of the shoulder blade (scapula).

Repeat for the other shoulder.

9 THUMB PUSHES

Place your hands on the receiver's shoulders, with your thumbs at the back and your fingers resting at the front of the shoulders.

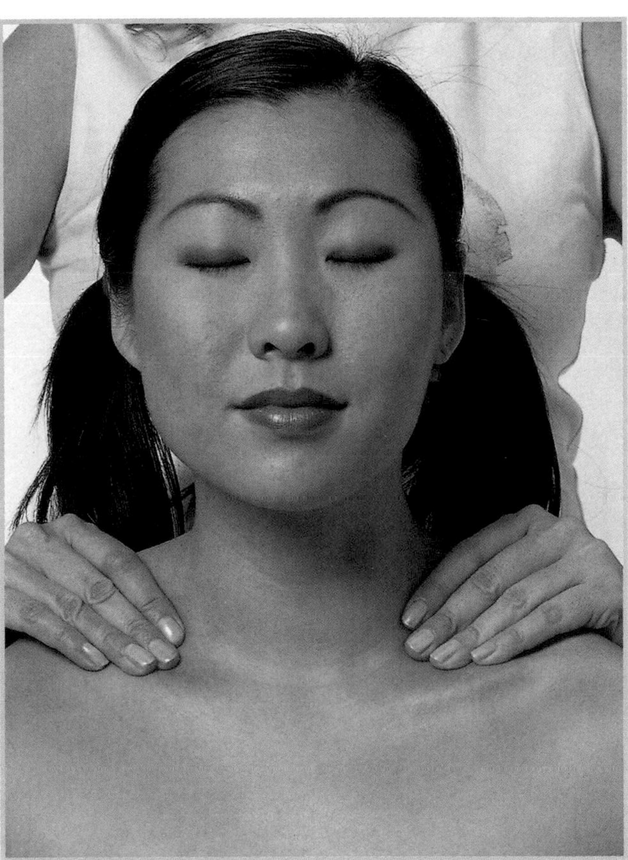

Push forwards with your thumbs towards your fingers, moving up and over the shoulder muscles. Try to pick up and squeeze as much muscle as you can as you work. Repeat these movements in the middle of the shoulders and also near the neck.

10 FINGER PULLS

i) After performing the thumb pushes in step 9, leave your hands on the receiver's shoulders.

Now, instead of rolling the muscle with your thumbs, use your fingers (which should be positioned at the front of the receiver's shoulders) to pull the muscle back towards your thumbs. Repeat the procedure in the middle of the shoulders and also near the neck.

11 PICKING UP AND SQUEEZING THE SHOULDER MUSCLES

Place the palm of each hand on top of each of the receiver's shoulders, with your thumbs positioned at the back and your fingers resting over the top of the shoulders.

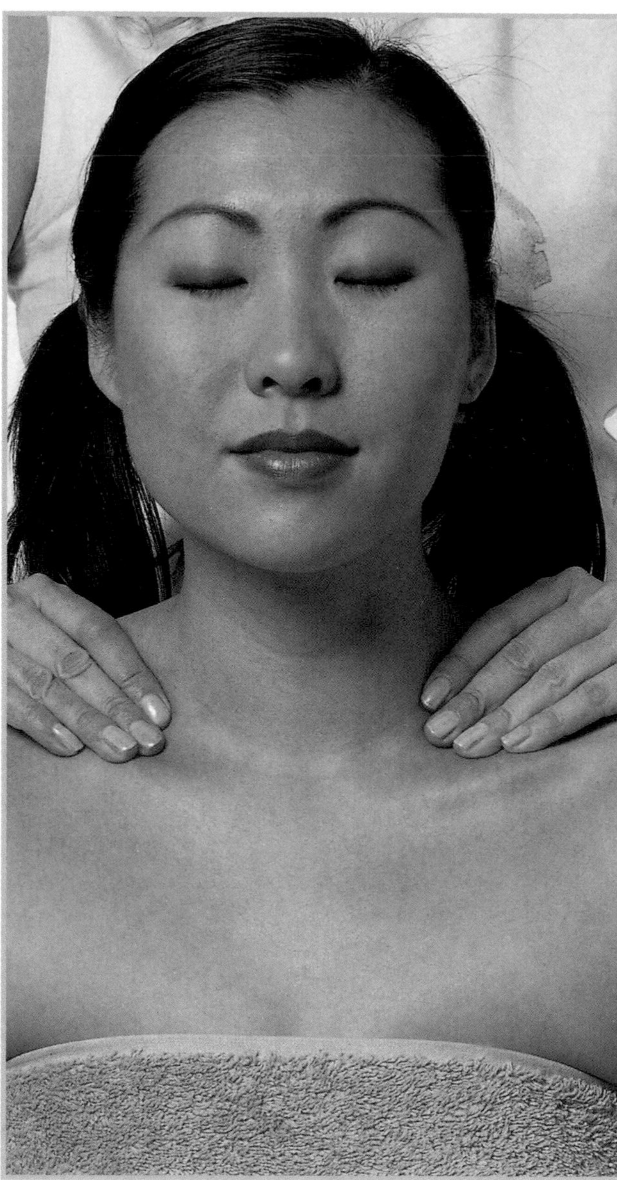

Using both hands, grasp the shoulder muscles firmly, pick them up, squeeze and then release them. It should feel as though you are sucking the shoulder muscles into the palms of your hands. If your partner has broad shoulders, place the palms of both hands on one shoulder to perform this technique.

12 SQUEEZING AND ROLLING THE SHOULDER MUSCLES

Stand behind the receiver and place the palms of your hands on each of their shoulders, with your fingers and thumbs at the front.

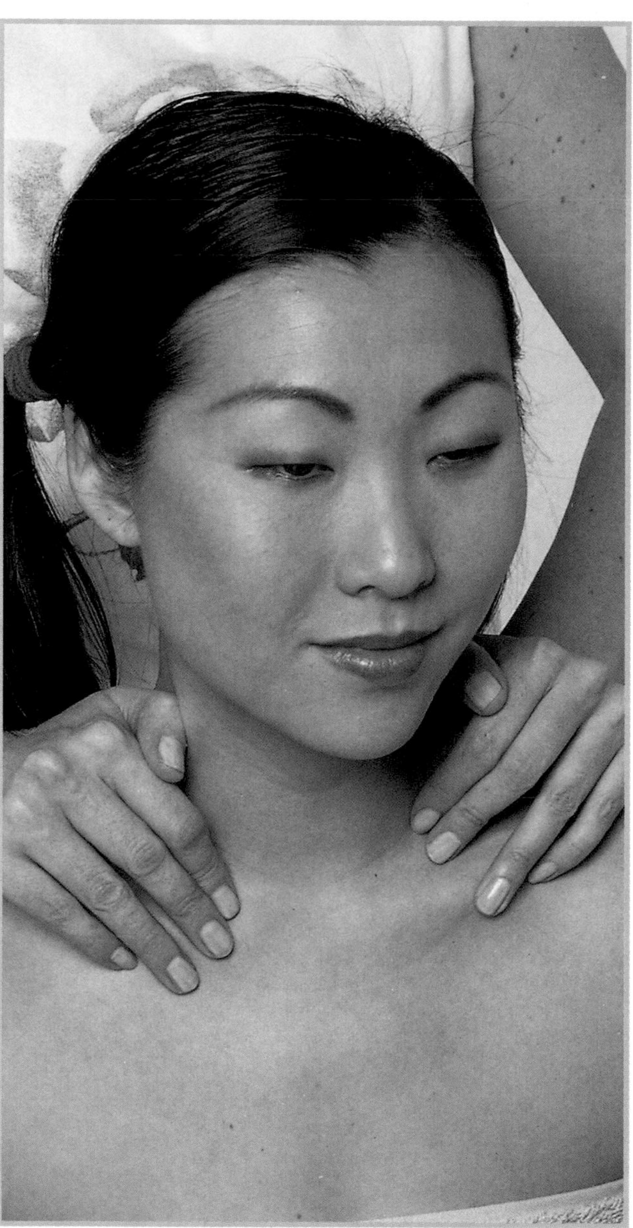

Press the heels of your hands into the back of the receiver's shoulders and gently roll the muscles forwards, over the top of the shoulders.

13 KNUCKLING THE SHOULDERS

Form your hands into fists and place your knuckles on each of the receiver's shoulders.

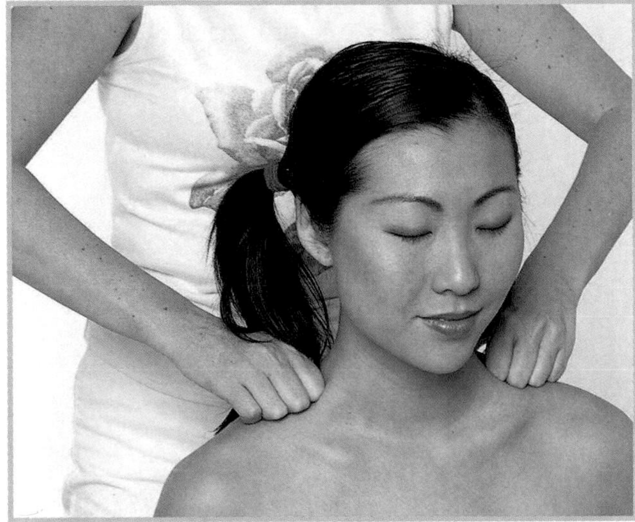

Now circle your knuckles across the top of your partner's shoulders, using a firm and steady pressure to loosen up the muscles.

14 WRINGING THE SHOULDERS

Place the palms of both hands on one of the receiver's shoulders.

Using one hand, pick up the muscle, squeeze and pull it towards you. Now repeat the process using the other hand. Using alternate hands, work rhythmically across the top of the shoulder.

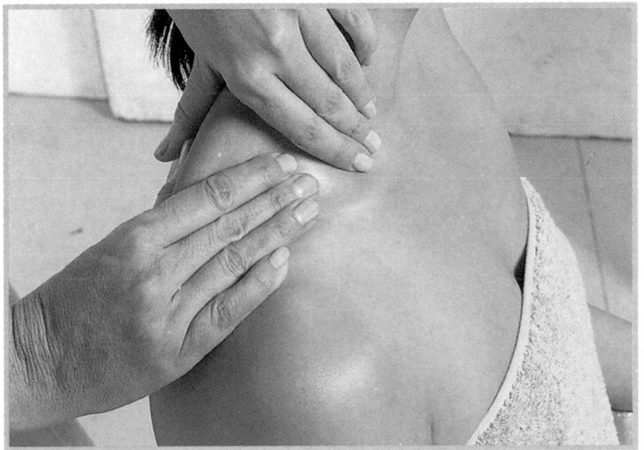

Repeat the procedure on the receiver's other shoulder.

15 CUPPING THE SHOULDERS

Now for the stimulating movements!

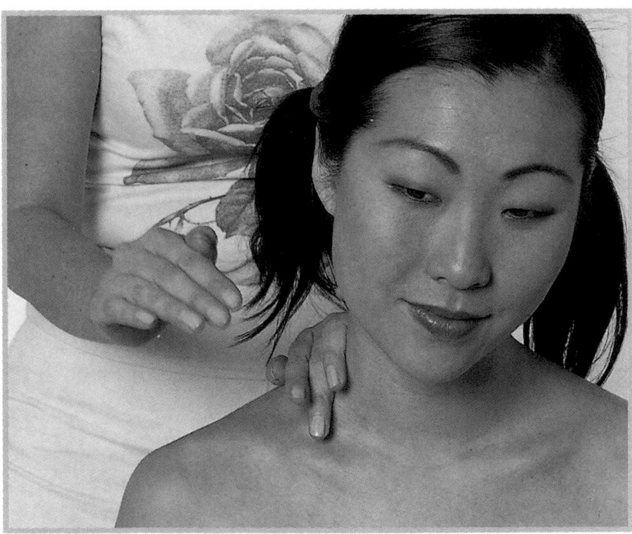

Form a hollow curve with both hands and bring your cupped hands down onto the receiver's shoulders in quick succession. Listen for the hollow sound.

16 HACKING THE SHOULDERS

First make sure that your wrists are loose. Then place your hands, with the palms facing each other and thumbs uppermost, over each of the receiver's shoulders.

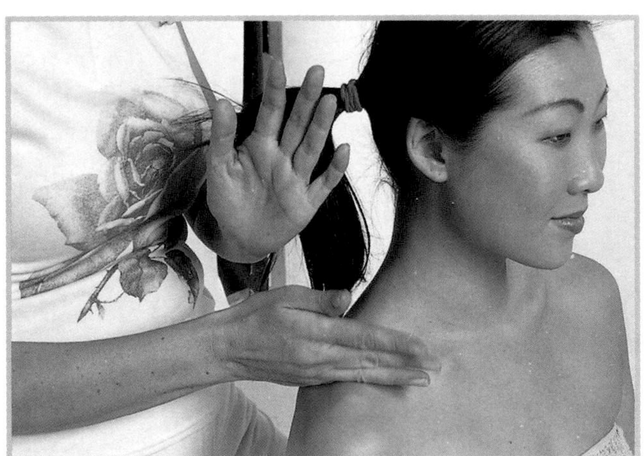

Flick your hands up and down in quick succession, allowing the edge of your hands to come into contact with the receiver's shoulders.

17 CHAMPIING THE SHOULDERS

Form your hands into a relaxed prayer position, so that only the heels of your hands and your fingertips remain in contact.

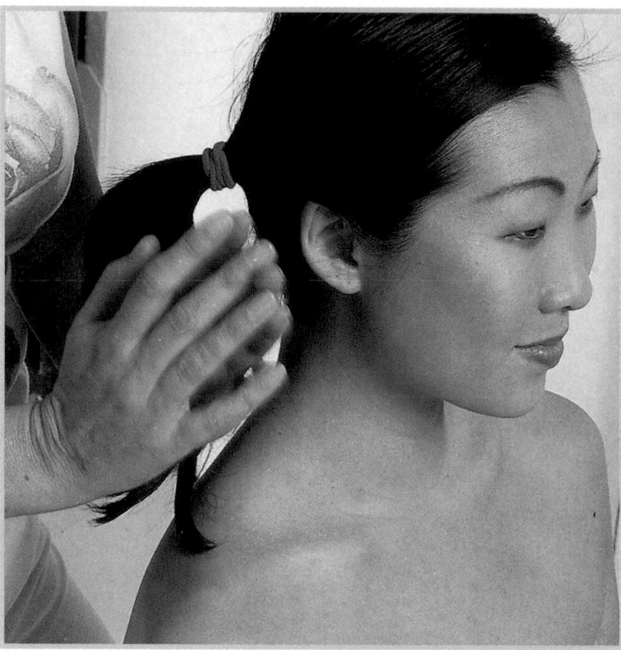

Now perform quick, light, striking movements across both of the receiver's shoulders with your 'cage' of fingers.

18 SMOOTHING THE SHOULDERS WITH THE FOREARMS

Stand behind the receiver. Form your hands into loose fists and then place one forearm on each of the receiver's shoulders, with your fists facing palm upwards.

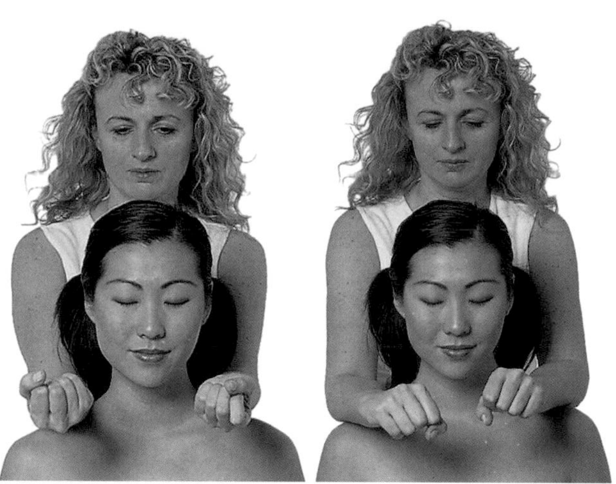

Now glide across your partner's shoulders with your forearms. As they glide, make a half-turn with your forearms so that your fists are facing palms downwards by the time that you reach the outside of the shoulders.

Repeat the procedure at least three times.

19 HOLDING THE SHOULDERS

To finish the upper-back and shoulder sequence, rest your hands very lightly on your partner's shoulders.

Feel the difference now that you have released the tension: the energy should now be flowing much more freely and the area should feel warm, supple and relaxed.

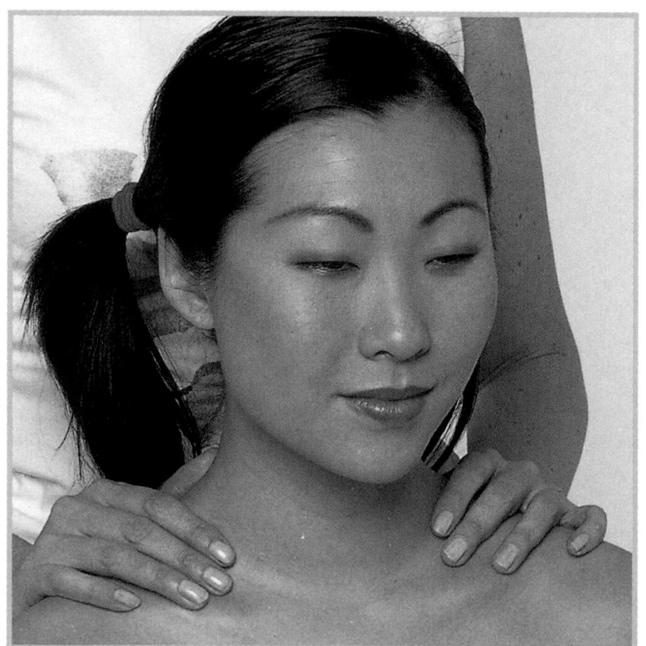

The upper arm sequence

1 STROKING DOWN, OR IRONING, THE SHOULDERS

Stand behind your partner and place one hand on each of their shoulders.

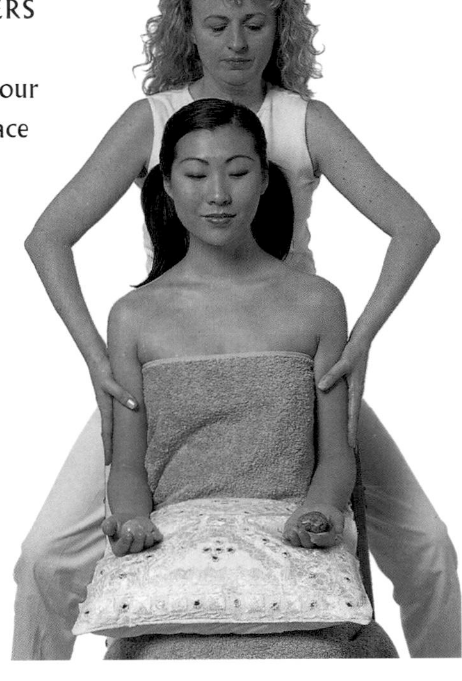

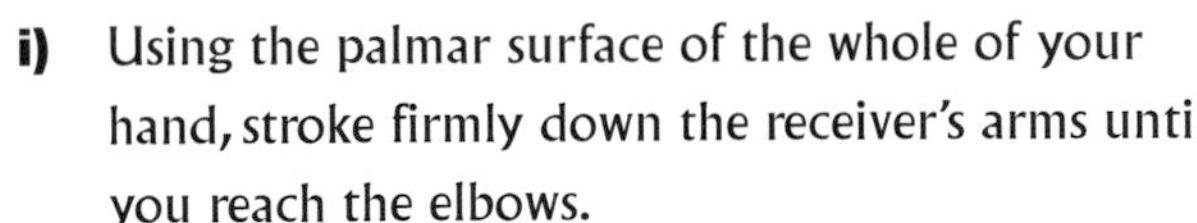

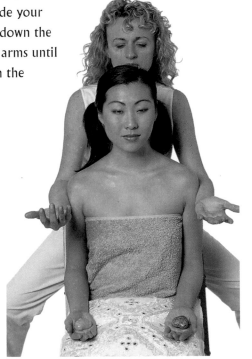

i) Using the palmar surface of the whole of your hand, stroke firmly down the receiver's arms until you reach the elbows. Repeat this movement several times, ensuring that you have covered the front, sides and back of the upper arms.

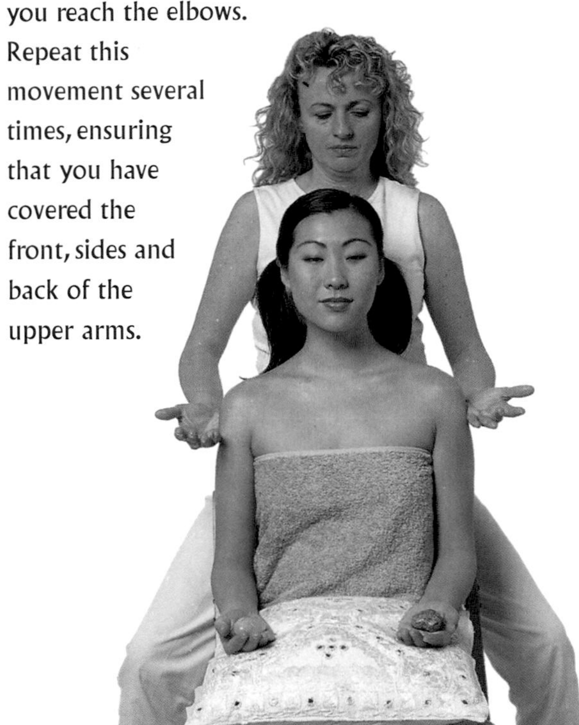

ii) You may also use the outer edge of your hands to perform this movement.

iii) For a really powerful action, slide your forearms down the receiver's arms until you reach the elbows.

2 SQUEEZING THE UPPER ARMS

Standing to one side of the receiver, place the palms of both of your hands around one of your partner's upper arms, one on the front and one on the back.

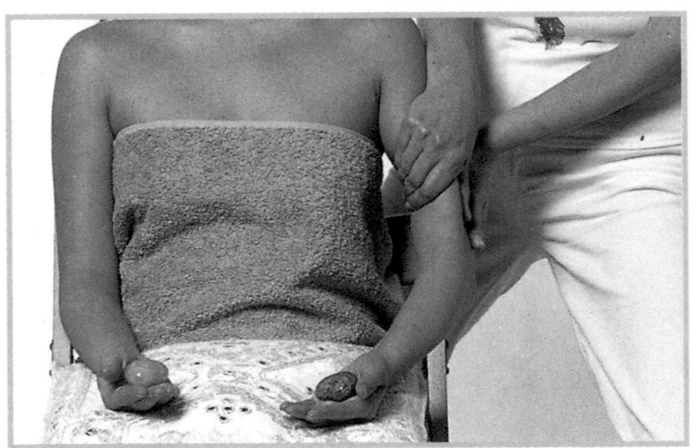

Gently squeeze and release the upper arm as you work down towards the elbow. Now glide your hands back up to your partner's shoulder. Repeat the procedure three times. Repeat the procedure on the other arm.

3 WRINGING THE UPPER ARMS

Stand to one side of the receiver.

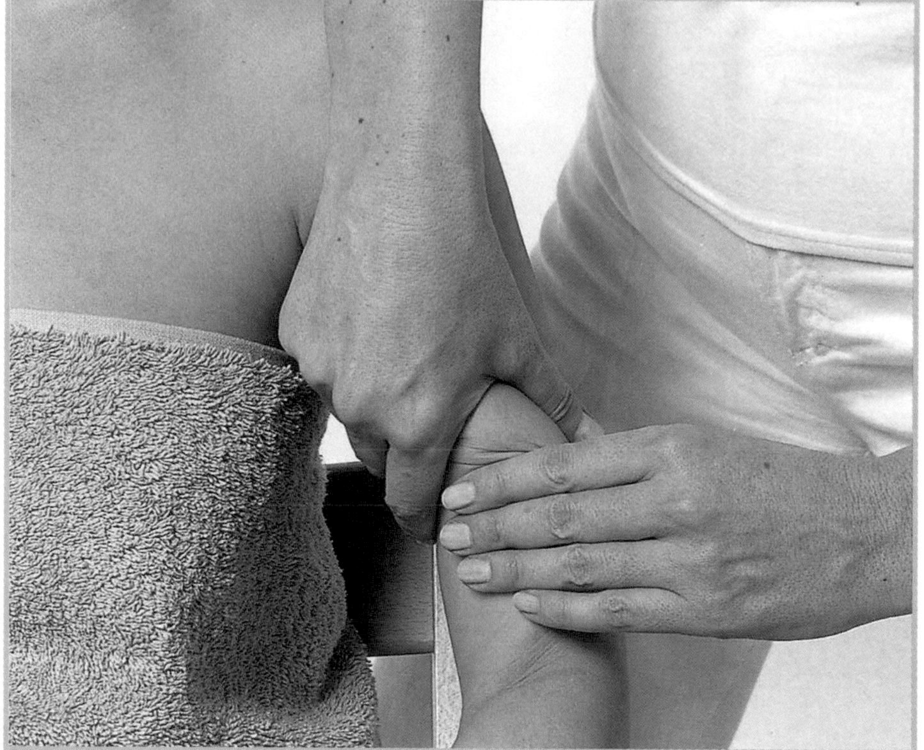

Place both of your hands on one of your partner's arms and, using alternate hands, rhythmically wring the upper arm, picking up as much muscle as you can. Repeat the procedure on the other arm.

4 HEEL ROLLING THE UPPER ARMS

Position your hands at the top of the receiver's upper arms, with your fingers in front and the heels of your hands behind.

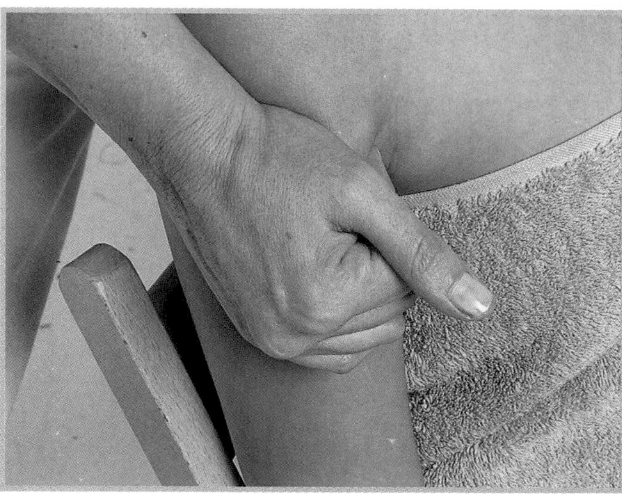

Roll the heels of your hands over the muscles until they meet your fingertips. Repeat the procedure in the middle of the upper arm and also just above the elbow. Heel roll each area at least three times.

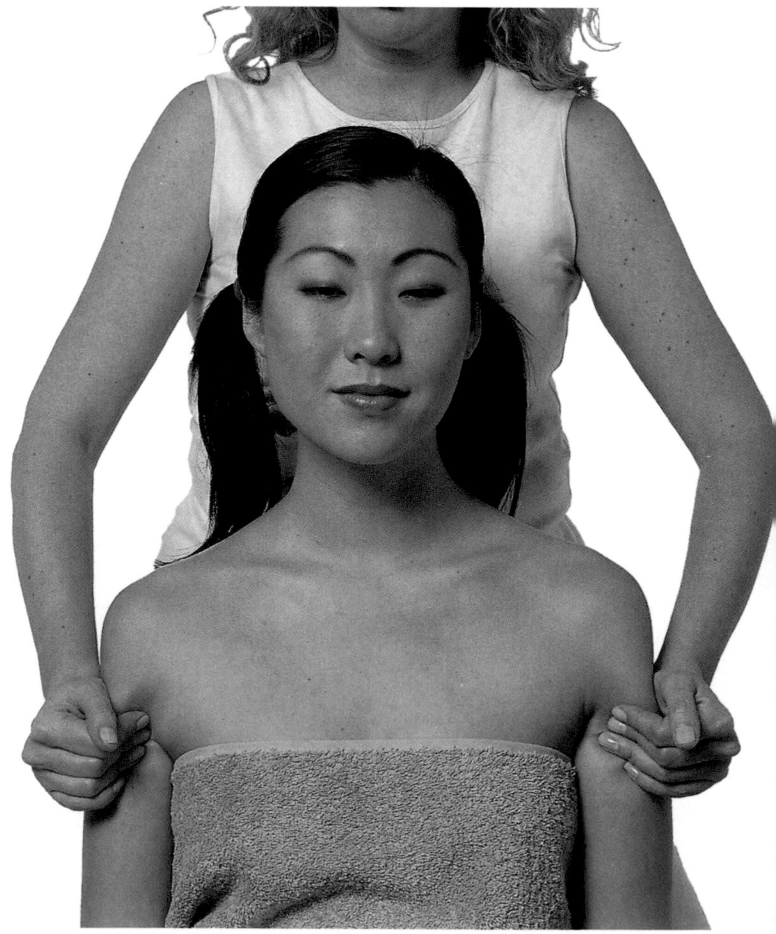

5 SHOULDER-LIFTING THE ARMS AND SHOULDERS

Stand behind the receiver and ask them to rest their hands in their lap.

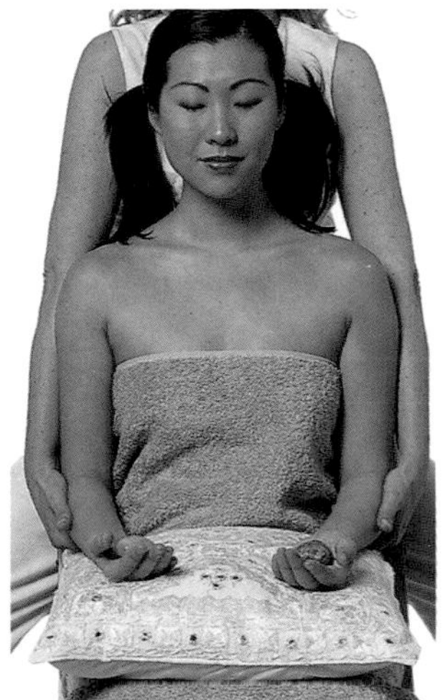

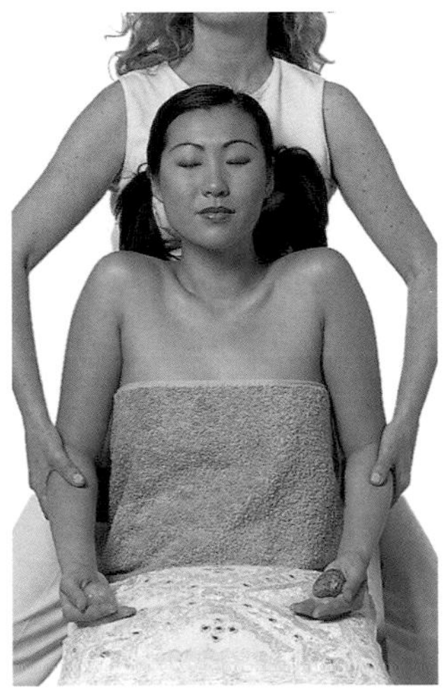

Place your hands under their elbows and then raise their arms and shoulders, holding the position for a few seconds before relaxing it. Repeat the procedure three times.

6 MOBILISING THE SHOULDERS

Position yourself at the receiver's side. Place one hand on one of their shoulders and the other under the elbow, supporting their hand in the crook of your elbow.

Gently move the shoulder both clockwise and anticlockwise. Repeat the procedure several times.

7 SMOOTHING THE UPPER ARMS

Stand behind the receiver.

Now, using the inside of your forearms, glide downwards along the receiver's upper arms. Repeat the procedure three times.

Using the palms of your hands, stroke downwards along the receiver's arms. Repeat the procedure three times.

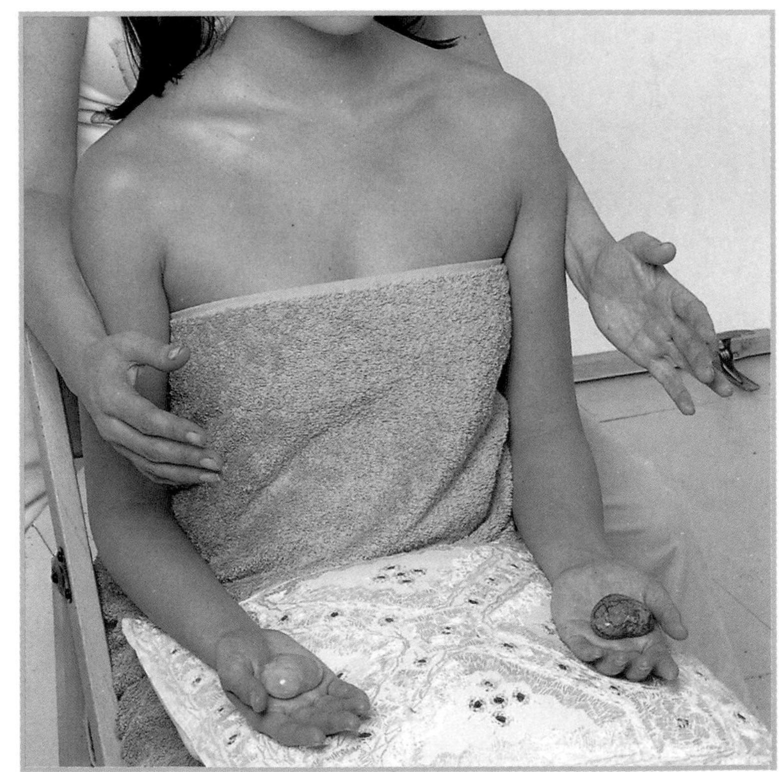

The neck sequence

1 ASSESSING THE TENSION IN THE NECK

Standing to the side of the receiver, place one hand on their forehead and one at the back of their neck.

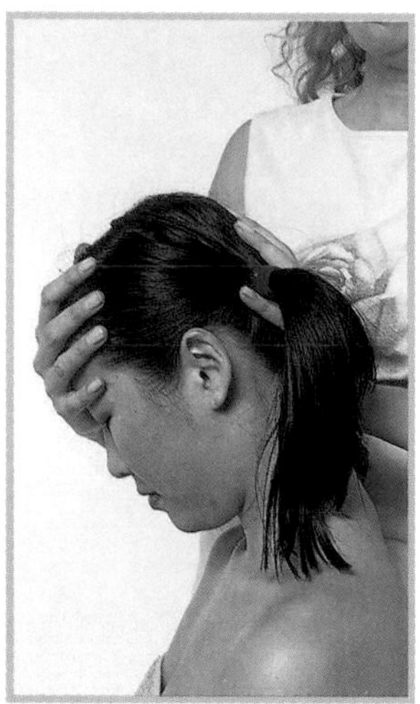

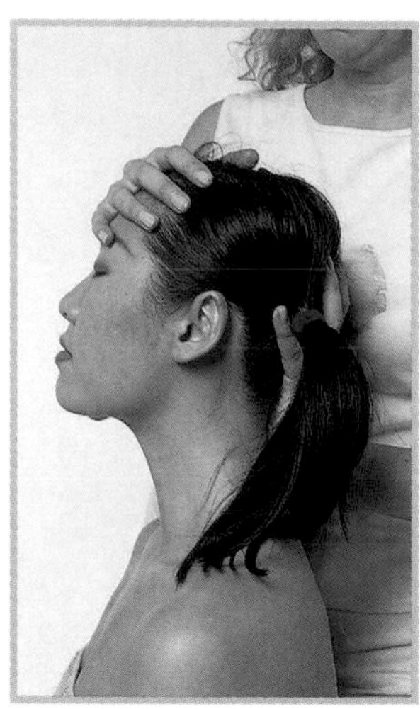

Now move your partner's head forwards and backwards very gently and slowly. Repeat the procedure three times.

2 KNEADING THE BACK OF THE NECK

Standing to the side of the receiver, gently place one hand on their forehead. Put the palm of your other hand on the bottom of the back of their neck, making a 'V' shape with your thumb and fingers.

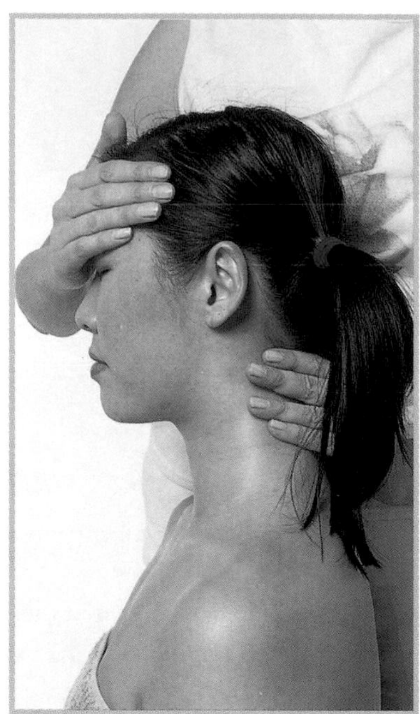

Pick up the muscles of the neck gently and slowly, repeating these movements as you work upwards until reaching the base of the skull. Then work from the base of the skull to the bottom of the neck.

3 FRICTIONING THE SIDE OF THE NECK

Standing behind and to the side, tilt the receiver's head gently to the side. Support their head by placing one hand on their forehead and then allowing their head to rest on your forearm.

Position the fingers of your other hand at the top of the neck and perform gentle, circular frictions as you work all the way down it. Repeat the procedure three times. Repeat the procedure on the other side of the neck.

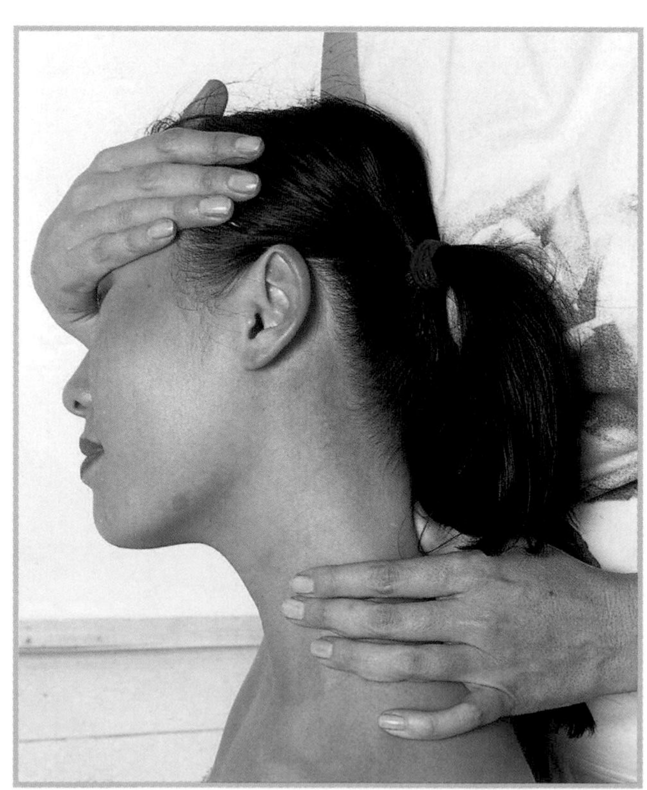

4 SQUEEZING AND RELEASING THE NECK

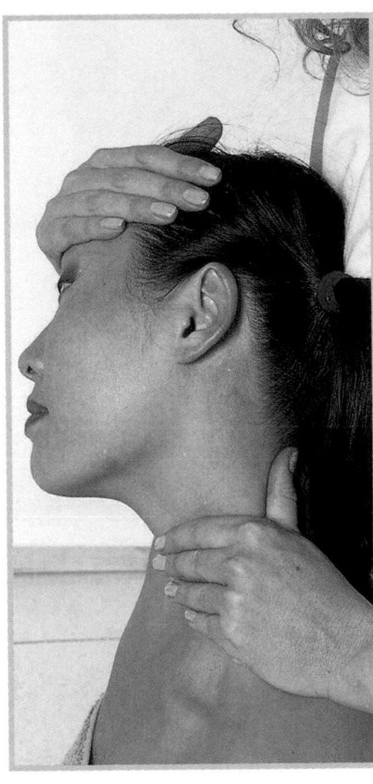

Tilt the receiver's head gently to the side. Support their head by placing one hand on their forehead and then allowing their head to rest on your forearm.

Now form a 'V' shape with the thumb and fingers of your other hand. Working gently and slowly, squeeze and release the muscles down the side of the neck. Repeat the procedure on the other side of the neck.

5 THUMB PUSHES TO THE SIDE OF THE NECK

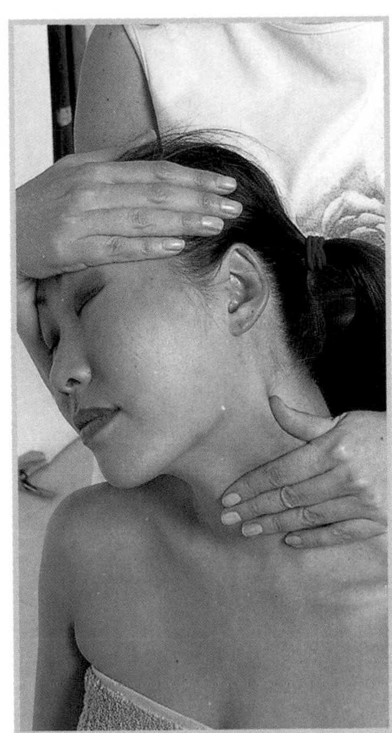

Tilt the receiver's head gently to the side. Support their head by placing one hand on their forehead and then allowing their head to rest on your forearm.

Starting under the ear, use the thumb of your other hand to push the muscles from the back of the neck gently towards the front. Repeat this movement down the entire length of the neck. Now perform these thumb pushes along the other side of the neck.

6 FINGER PULLS TO THE SIDE OF THE NECK

Tilt the receiver's head gently to the side. Support their head by placing one hand on their forehead and then allowing their head to rest on your forearm.

Starting under the ear, instead of pushing your thumb forwards, this time gently draw your fingers back towards your thumb. Repeat this movement down the entire length of the neck. Repeat this technique on the other side of the neck.

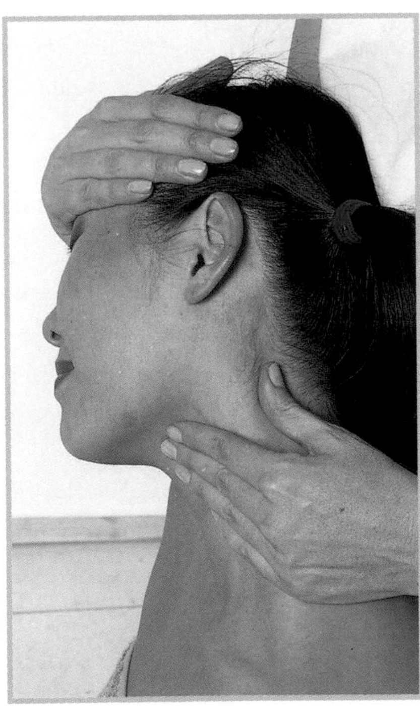

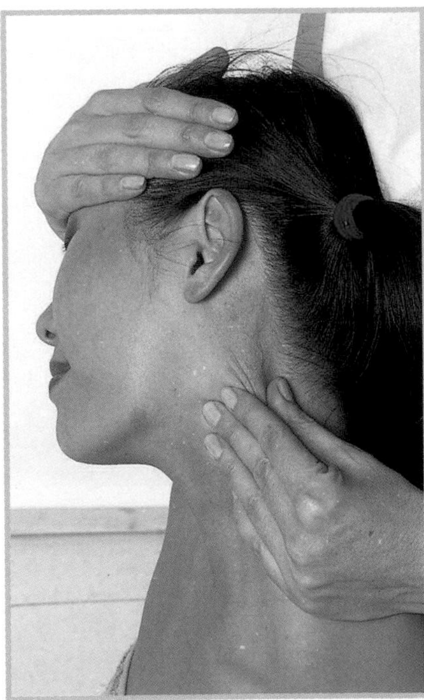

7 HEEL RUBBING UNDER THE BASE OF THE SKULL

Stand to the side of the receiver. Place one hand over their forehead to give support and tilt their head forwards very slightly.

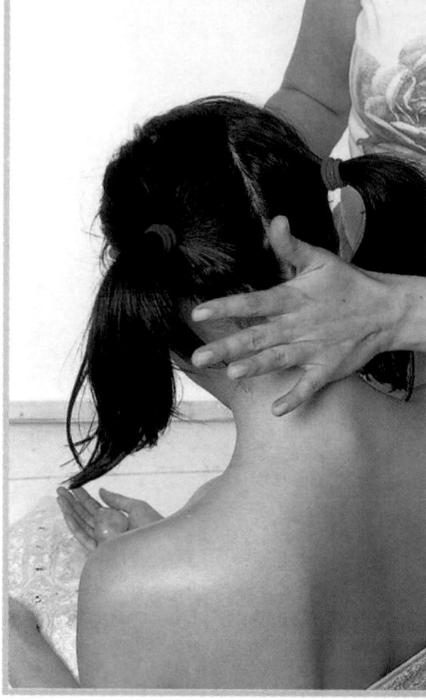

Position the heel of your other hand at the base of the skull (occiput) and then rub lightly and briskly over the area.

9 STROKING DOWN THE NECK

Stand to the side of the receiver and place one hand over their forehead to give support. Using your other hand, gently stroke down the back and sides of the receiver's neck to remove any residual tension.

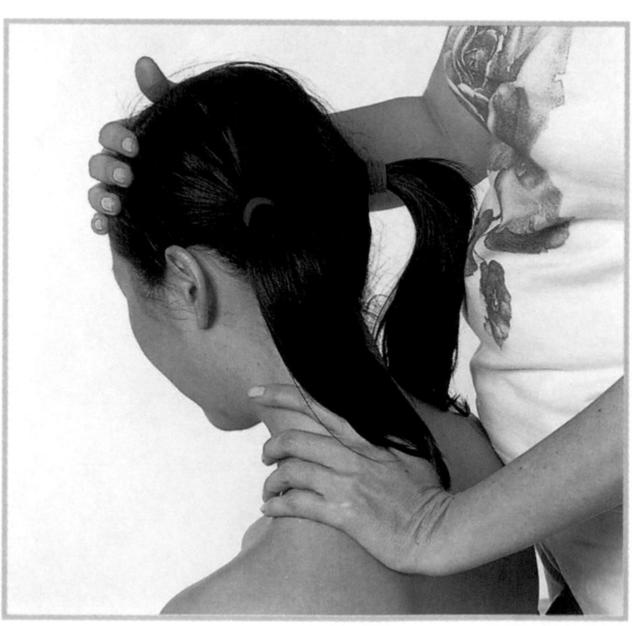

8 FRICTIONING UNDER THE BASE OF THE SKULL

Stand to the side of the receiver. Place one hand over their forehead to give support and tilt their head backwards very slightly.

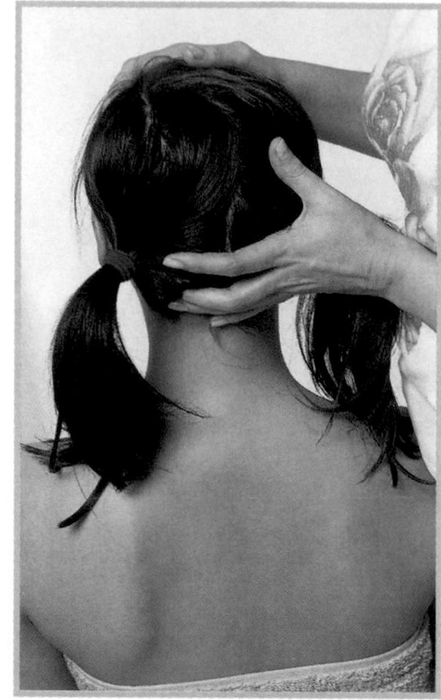

Position the pads of the fingers of your other hand at the base of the skull (occiput). Gently friction along the skull, working from one ear to the other.

The scalp sequence

NB:
If the receiver's hair has been clipped or tied up, out of the way, this is the point when you should remove the clip or tie.

1 CONNECTING WITH THE SCALP

Gently place your hands on either side of the receiver's head. Hold this position until you feel connected with your partner. Try to become aware of how much tension is being held in the scalp.

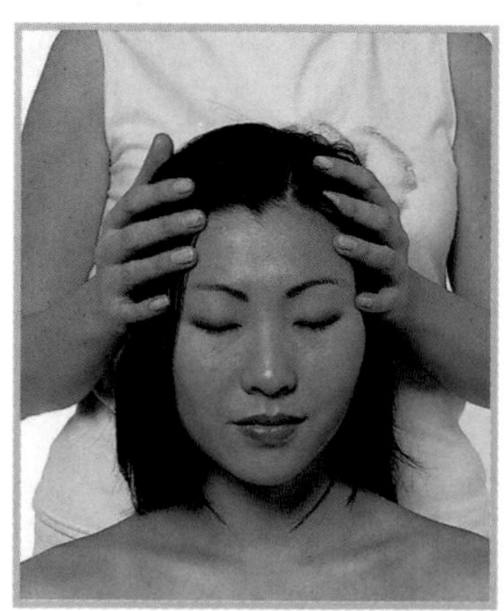

2 RUBBING THE SIDE OF THE SCALP

Stand behind, or slightly to the side of, the receiver. Gently place one hand on one of your partner's temples, with your fingers resting on their forehead to support their head.

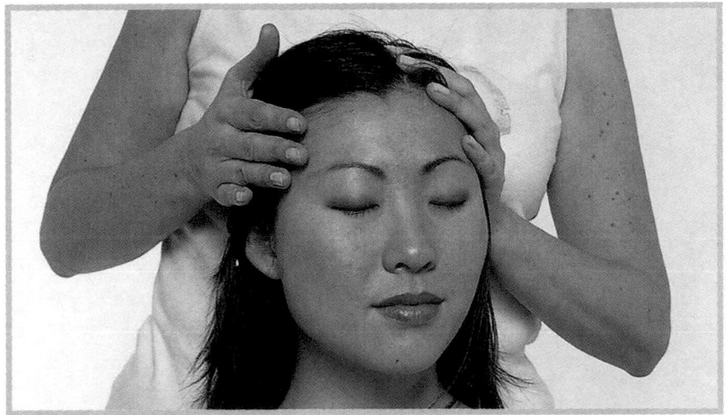

Place your other hand on the other side of the receiver's head and use your palm to rub it briskly, working from the top of the neck to behind the ear and then up towards the crown of the head. Your hand should be moving rapidly back and forth up the side of the head and then back down again.

3 RUBBING THE TOP OF THE HEAD

Standing behind the receiver, gently support their head with one hand. Place your other hand on the crown of your partner's head, with your fingers facing forwards.

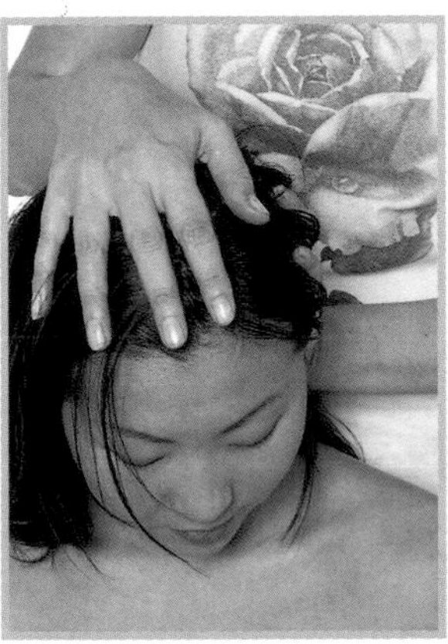

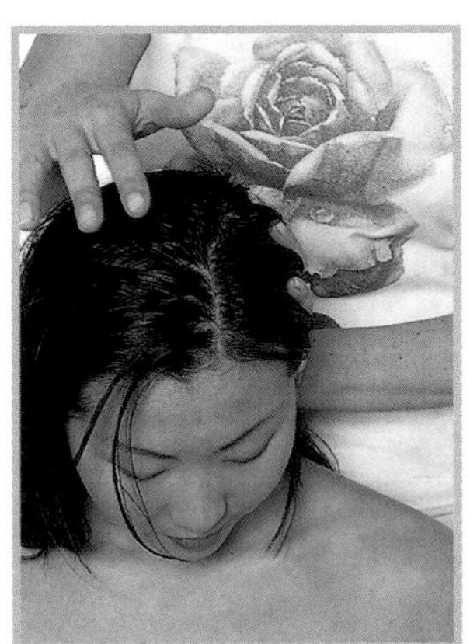

Using your whole hand, work with a zigzag, side-to-side action from the front of the scalp to the back, and then from the back to the front again. Repeat the procedure several times, making yourself aware of the movement of the scalp.

4 WHOLE HAND FRICTIONING

Stand behind the receiver and place your hands on either side of their head. (If you wish, you could gently rest the receiver's head against your body to provide extra support).

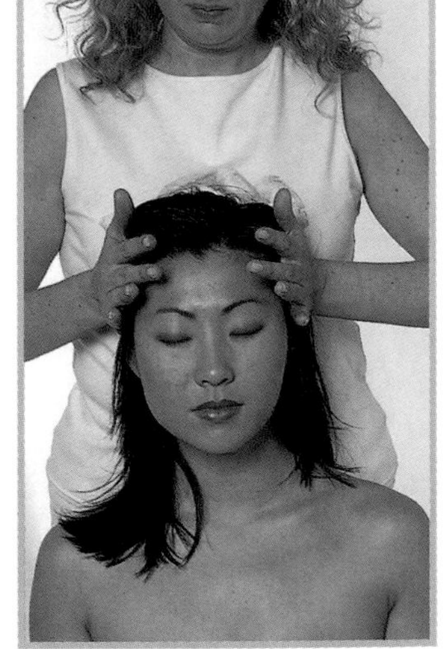

Use the heels of your hands to circle up and down the sides, top and back of the scalp, working gradually and applying firm, yet gentle, pressure.

5 FINGER PAD FRICTIONING OR 'SHAMPOOING' THE SCALP

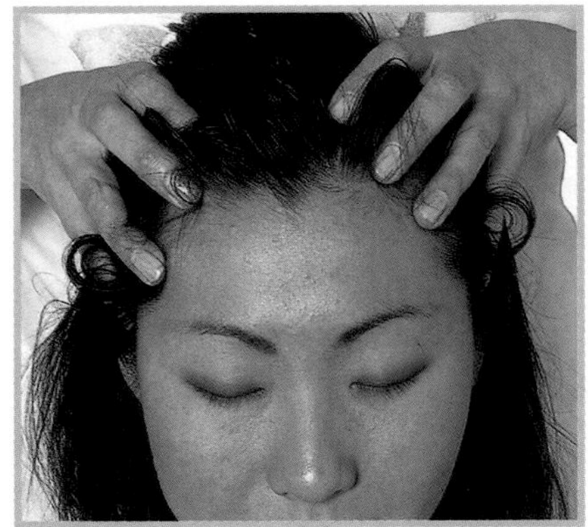

Form your hands into claw-like shapes and then gently rest them on the sides of the receiver's head.

Spread out your fingers and then, using your finger pads, perform small, slow, circular movements over the whole of the scalp. Your pressure should be fairly firm as you 'shampoo' the scalp. As you work, you should feel the scalp starting to move more freely as the tension is released.

6 RUFFLING THE HAIR

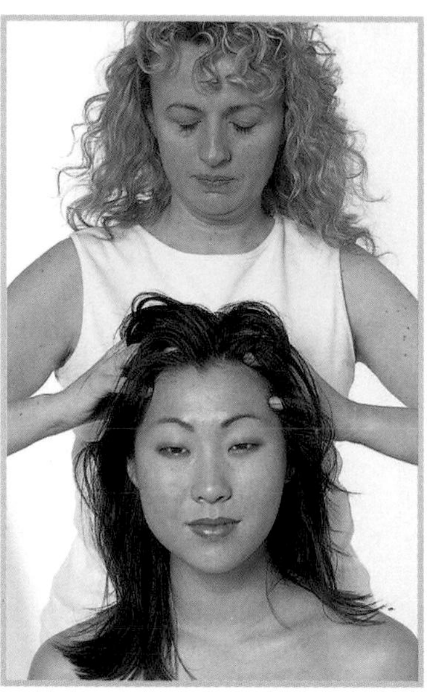

Spread out your fingers and then rest your hands on the receiver's scalp.

Using the pads of your fingers, gently ruffle your partner's entire head of hair, keeping your wrists loose and relaxed. (You may find it easier to support the receiver's head with one hand and to ruffle the hair with the other.)

7 PLUCKING THE HAIR

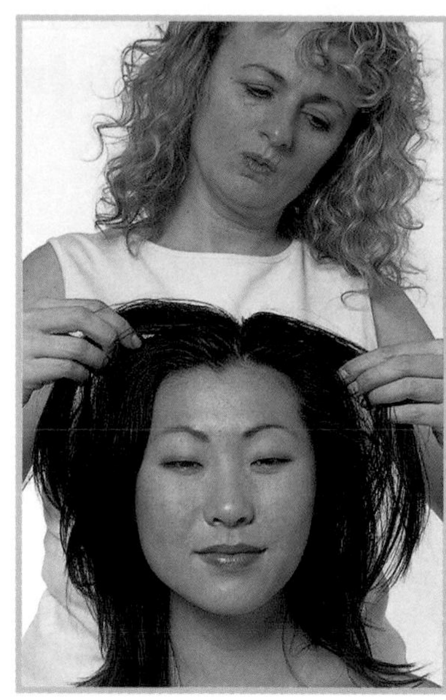

Form your hands into loose claw shapes, spread out your fingers and then place them gently on the receiver's head.

Bring your fingers and thumbs together as you lift them away from the head, gathering up small amounts of hair as you work across the entire scalp. If you wish, you could give the hair a gentle tug to stimulate growth.

8 TABLA PLAYING OR TAPPING THE SCALP

Hold your hands above the receiver's scalp and then use two fingertips gently to tap (or drum) all over the receiver's head.

As your fingertips bounce off the hair, the action should resemble raindrops falling to the ground. Try tapping the receiver's scalp with all of your fingertips, as well as only two.

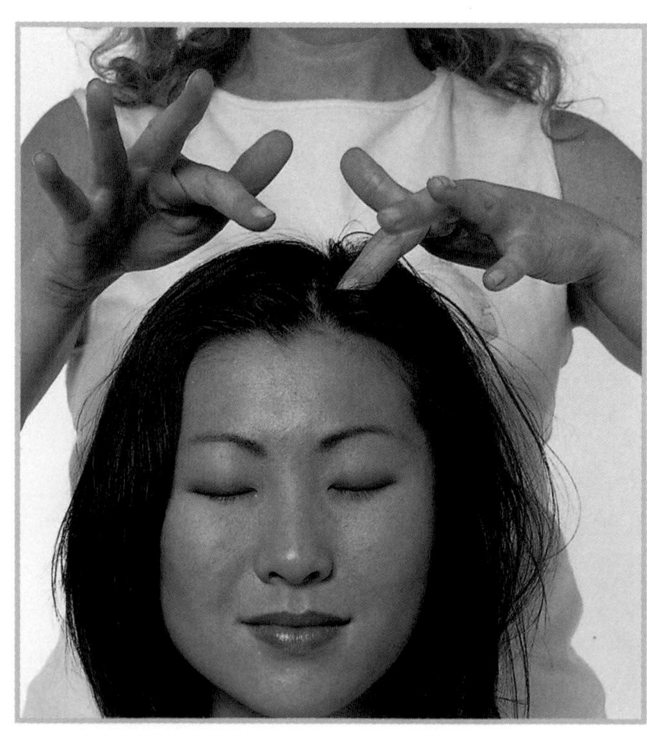

9 STROKING OR 'COMBING THROUGH' THE HAIR

Standing behind the receiver, rest both of your hands on their head, with your fingers facing forwards.

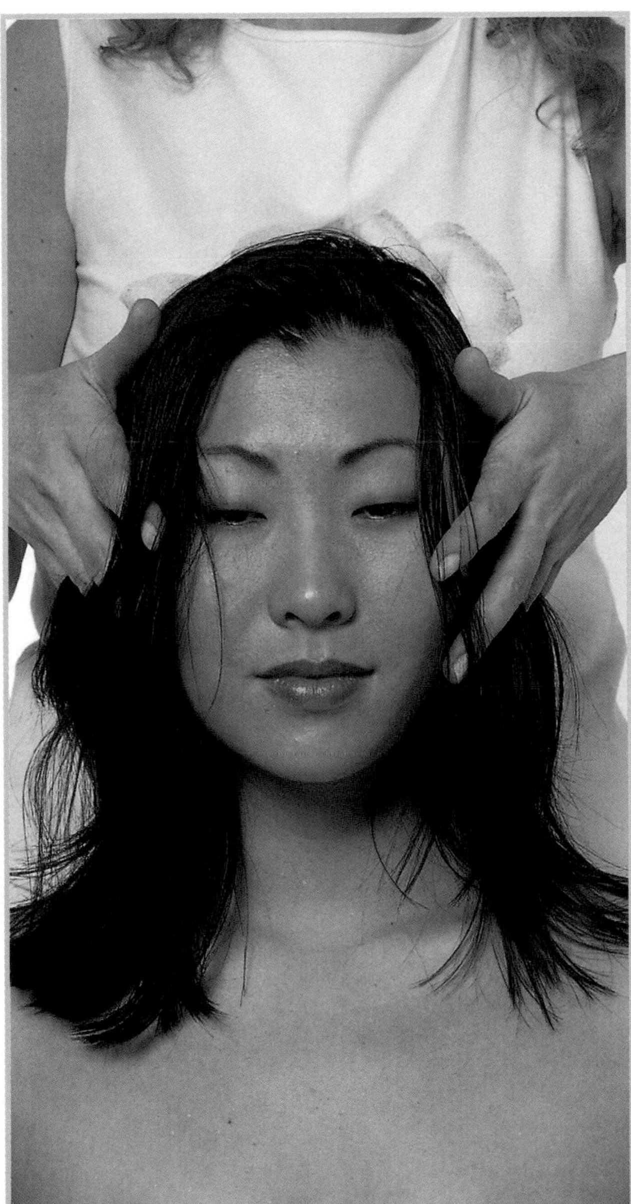

Use the fingertips of alternate hands gently to stroke down the length of your partner's head. As one hand finishes, the other hand should start, so that it feels like one continuous movement. This is an extremely relaxing technique, but if the receiver requires stimulating, you could use your fingernails, taking care, of course, not to scratch your partner.

The facial sequence

NB:

To perform the facial massage sequence, place a rolled-up towel or pillow behind the receiver's neck. Then allow their head to rest gently against your body.

1 STROKING THE FACE

Place the palms of your hands, with your fingers interlocking, on the receiver's forehead.

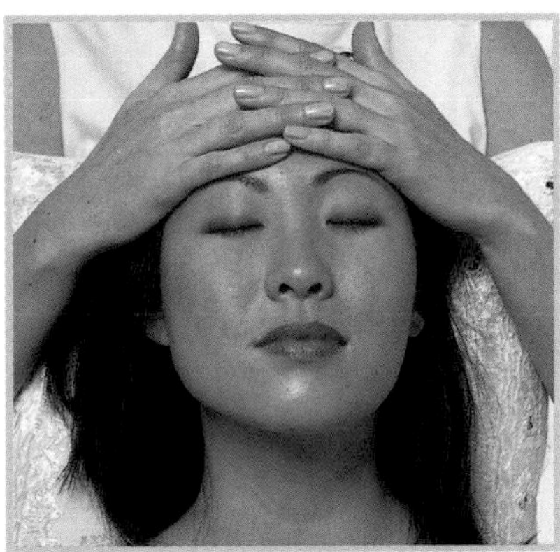

i) Now gently draw your hands apart, stroking outwards, across the forehead towards the temples. Using no pressure, glide your hands back to your starting position. Repeat the procedure several times.

ii) Alternatively, place one hand on the receiver's forehead and then stroke across their face, towards the temples. As this hand finishes, repeat the stroking procedure with the other hand. Both techniques are wonderfully relaxing.

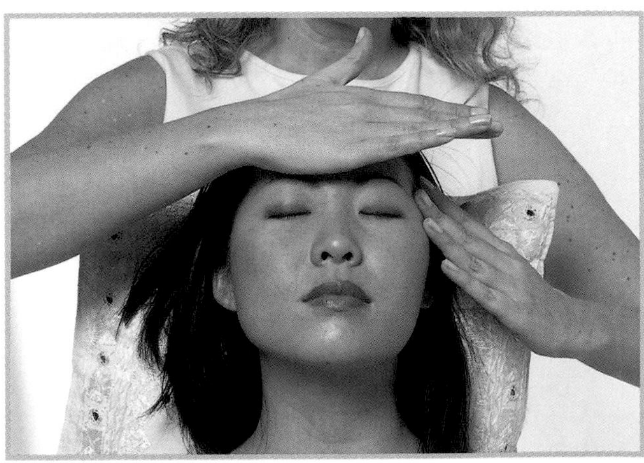

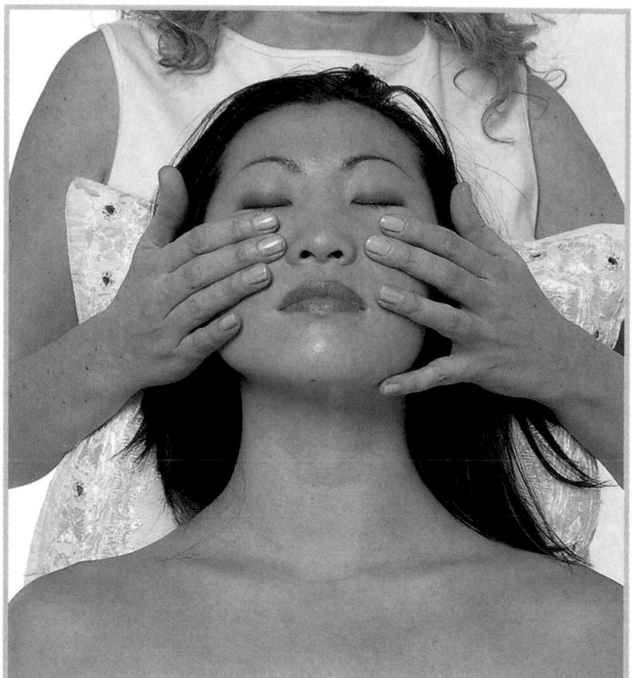

iii) Place a hand on each of the receiver's cheeks and then stroke outwards, across the cheeks towards the ears. Repeat the procedure several times.

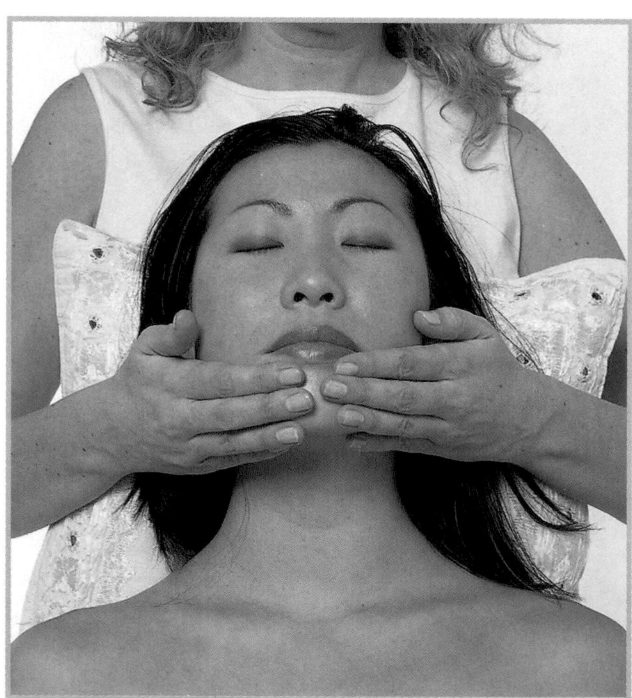

iv) Now place your hands in the centre of the receiver's chin. Using both hands, stroke outwards, across the face, moulding your hands to fit the contours of the chin.

2 PRESSING AND RELEASING THE FACIAL PRESSURE POINTS

Place the pads of your thumbs in the centre of the receiver's forehead, just below the hairline.

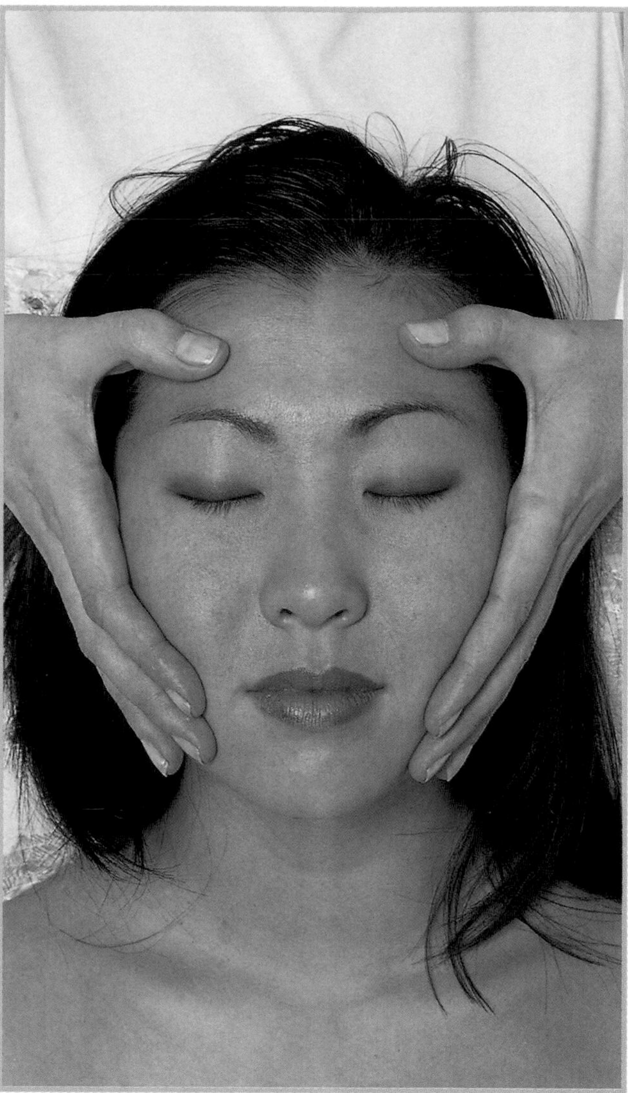

i) Working outwards in a horizontal row, gently press and release the pressure points at intervals of one to two centimetres. After completing the first row, bring your thumbs back to the centre of the forehead, but place them slightly lower down. Repeat another row of pressure points. Continue pressing and releasing in horizontal rows until you reach the receiver's eyebrows. If you wish, you could use the pads of your index or middle fingers instead.

ii) Place the pads of your index or middle fingers next to the receiver's nose, just below the eyes. Gently pressing and releasing, work outwards across the cheeks, following the line of the cheekbones. Continue working in horizontal strips as you did for the forehead until you reach the receiver's mouth.

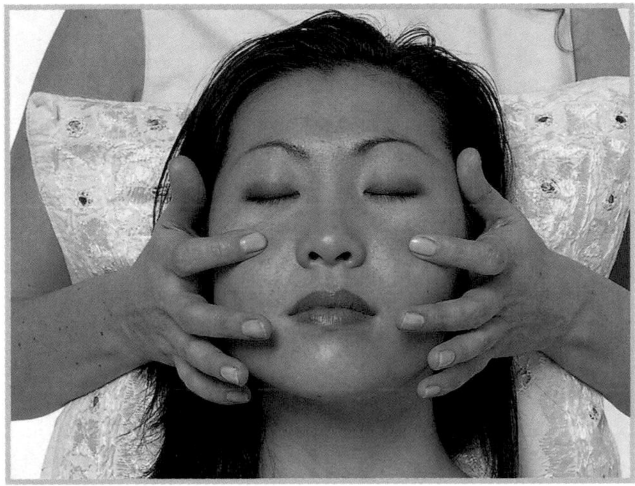

NB:
Working across the forehead and cheek area may help to clear the sinuses.

iii) Repeat the pressing-and-releasing procedure on the receiver's chin, commencing in the centre of the chin,
just below the mouth, and working in horizontal rows until you reach the bottom of the chin.

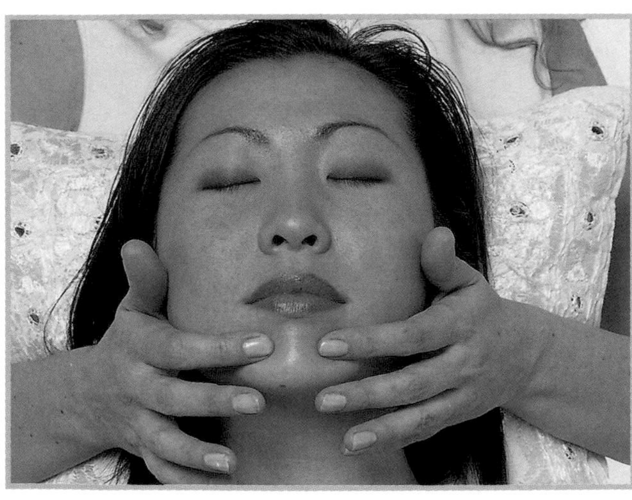

3 RELEASING JAW TENSION

Lightly cup the receiver's jaw between the thumbs and index fingers of both of your hands.

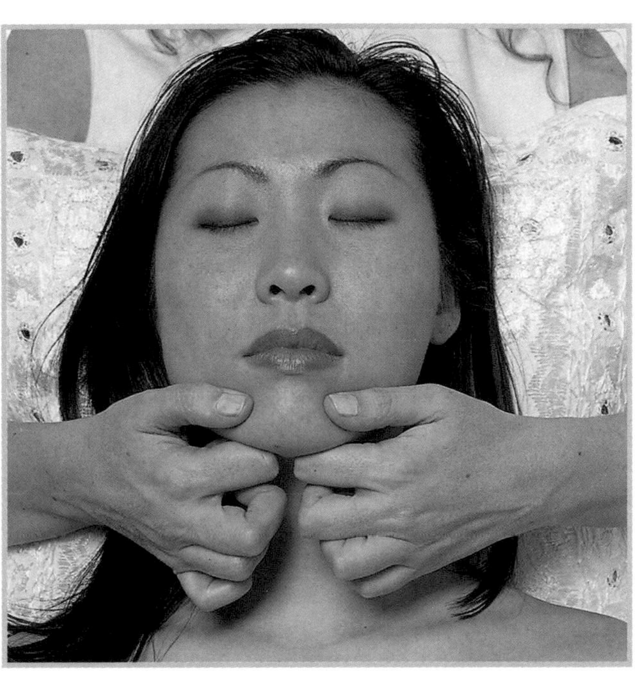

i) Gently squeeze the flesh between your thumbs and index fingers.

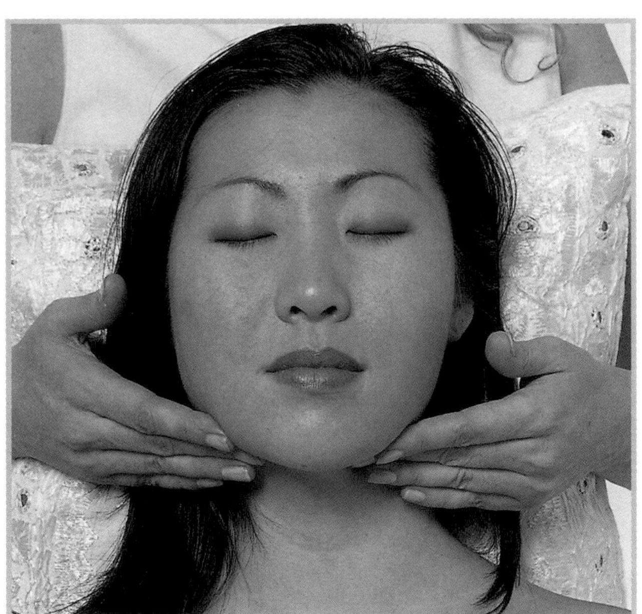

ii) Place the pads of your index and middle fingers under the centre of the jaw and perform circular friction along the jaw line until you reach the ears.

4 MASSAGING THE EARS

Position yourself behind the receiver and place the palms of your hands over each of their ears.

i) Using very light pressure and a circular motion, work your palms over all of the ear area.

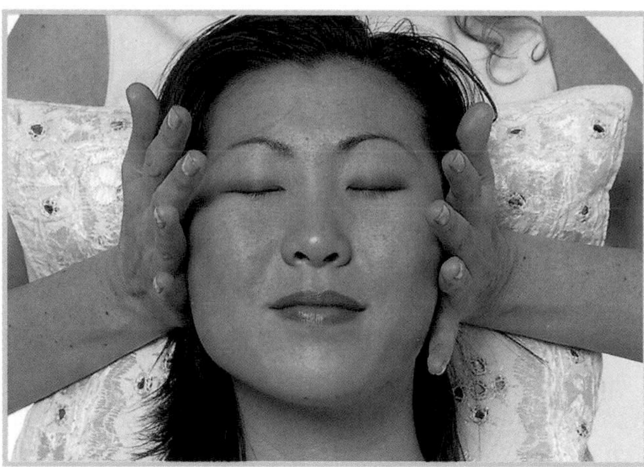

ii) Beginning with the earlobes, gently squeeze the skin between your thumbs and forefingers. Work up and down the ears, gently massaging and squeezing them.

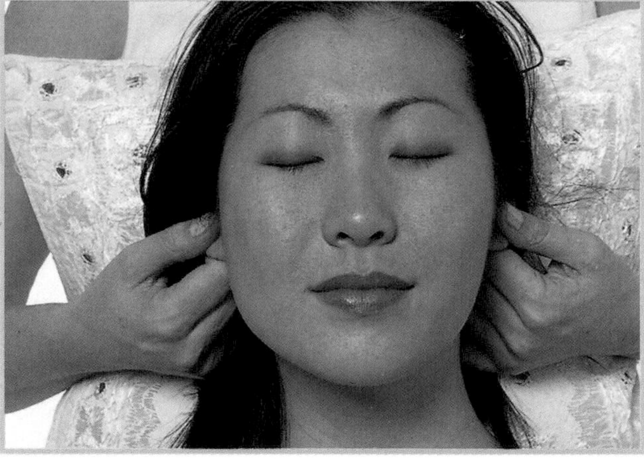

NB:
Massaging the ears will benefit all of the body's systems, while applying acupressure to the ear can be used to treat many disorders of the body and mind.

5 CIRCULAR TEMPLE-FRICTIONING

Position your fingers over the receiver's temples.

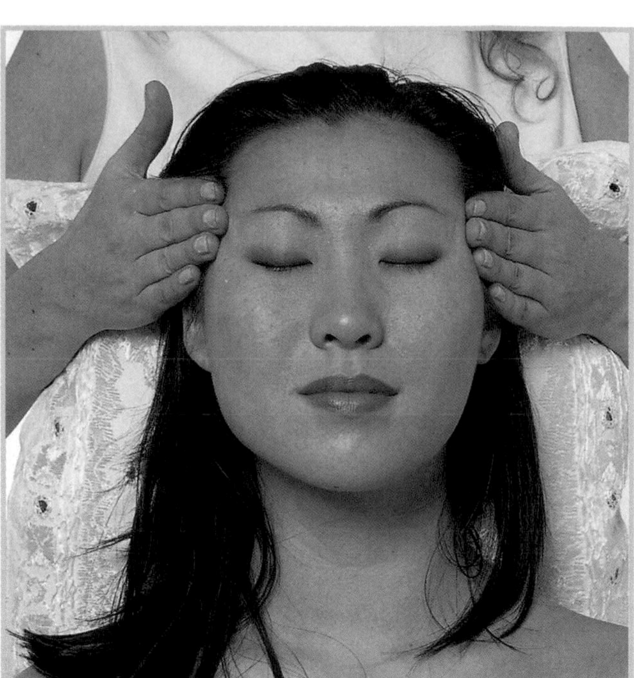

i) Using slow, circular movements and very gentle pressure, massage the temple areas with the pads of your fingers.

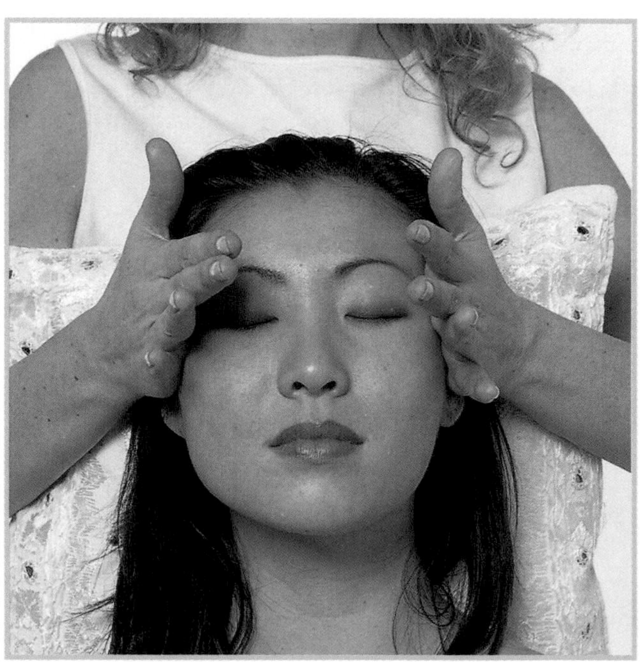

ii) For a deeper action, perform this movement with the heels of your hands.

6 FACIAL-TAPPING

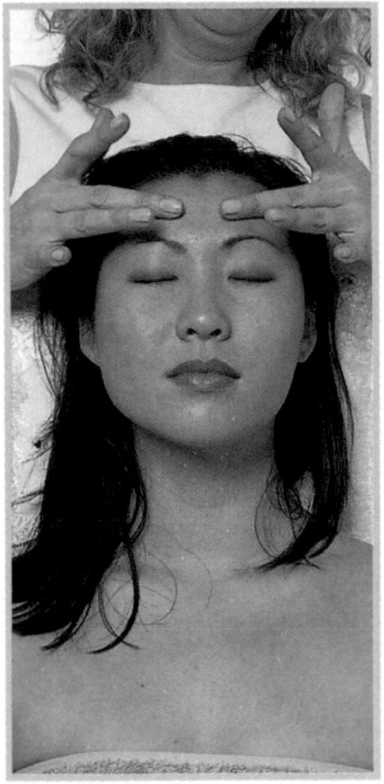

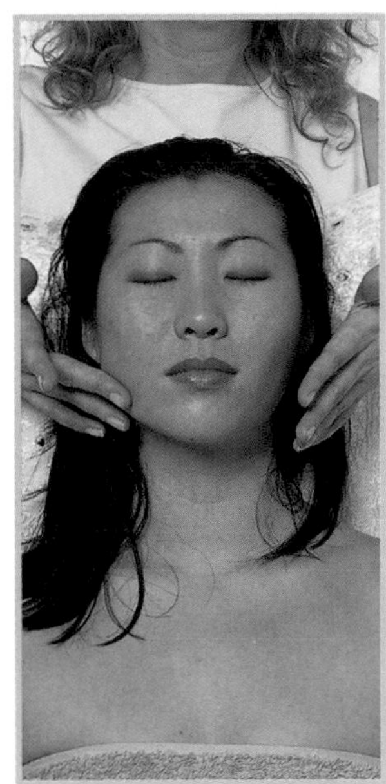

With a light touch, use the pads of your fingers to tap over all of your partner's face, as well as under their chin.

7 FEATHER-LIKE FINGERTIP STROKING

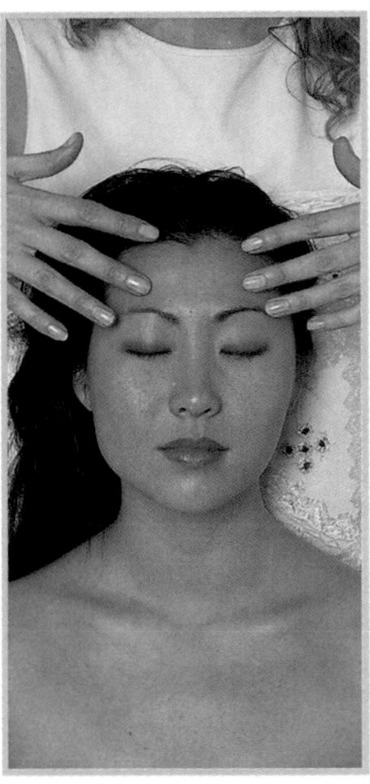

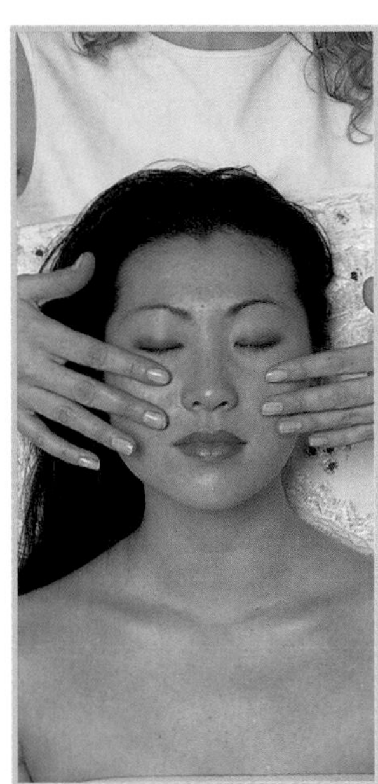

Using the pads of your fingers and a feather-light touch, gently stroke across the receiver's forehead, cheeks and chin. Do this several times.

8 THE FINAL TOUCH

To complete the facial sequence, gently rest your hands on your partner's head. Hold this position for about thirty seconds before gradually releasing your hands.

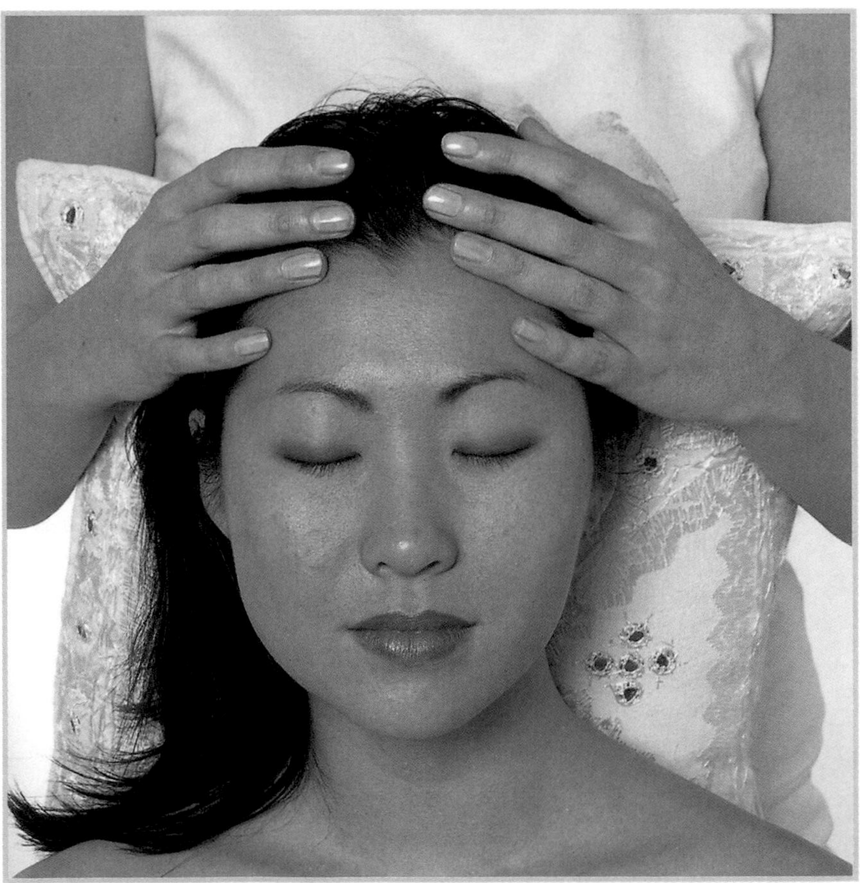

The chakra balancing sequence

Chakra balancing is described in detail between pages 55 and 56. Refer to Chapter 4 for more information on chakras.

1 GROUNDING YOURSELF

Position yourself at the receiver's side. Ensure that you feel grounded by visualising roots extending from your feet deep into the earth.

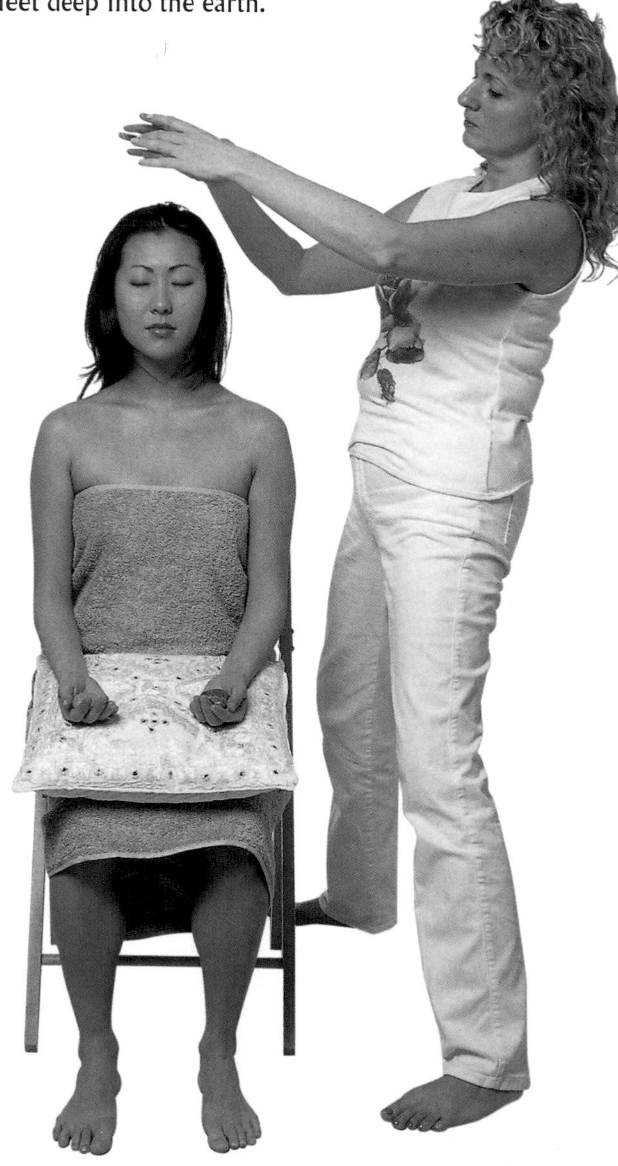

Allow your hands to hover just above your partner's head and then slowly glide them down your partner's body, without touching it, until you reach the base of the spine.

2 VISUALISING THE CHAKRAS

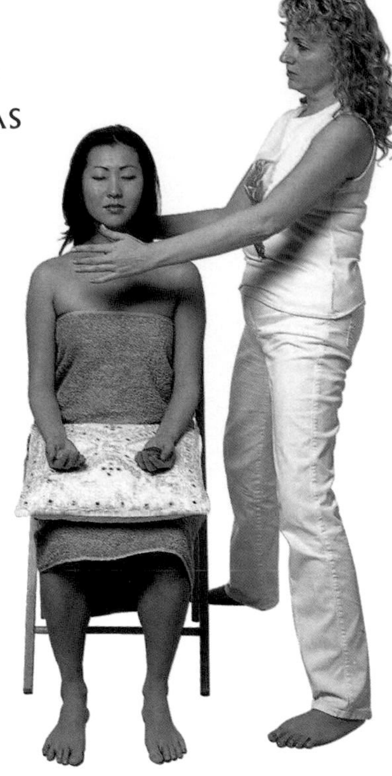

i) With the palms of your hands hovering a few centimetres away from the base chakra, visualise a clear, deep-red colour emanating from this energy centre.

ii) Move up to the sacral chakra and visualise a clear, orange colour.

iii) Move up to the solar plexus chakra and visualise a radiant golden light.

iv) Rise to the heart chakra and visualise a flower of pink light.

v) Move up to the throat chakra and visualise a blue light. (Chakra illustrated).

vi) Move up to the brow chakra and visualise an indigo-blue light.

vii) Rise to the crown chakra and visualise a bright, clear, violet light.

viii) Allow the receiver to bathe in the feelings of peace and relaxation that your Indian head massage has imparted.

3 GROUNDING THE RECEIVER

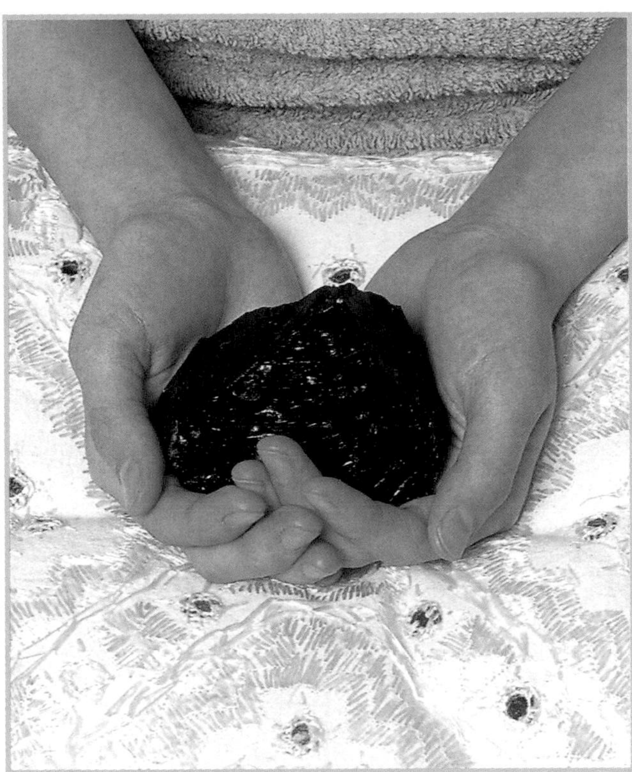

i) Move in front of your partner and place your hands on their feet. Rub them gently to ground the receiver.

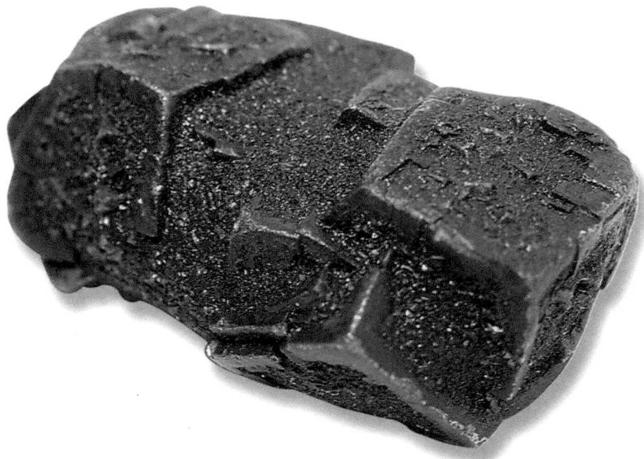

ii) If the receiver still feels slightly 'spacy', you could offer them a grounding stone, such as black tourmaline, smoky quartz, haematite, obsidian or a Boji™ stone, to hold.

iii) Allow the receiver to sit quietly for a minute or so while you wash your hands. Encourage them to drink a glass of water after the treatment and to put on a warm jumper or cardigan. If you have used oil on their hair, advise them to leave it on for a few hours in order to receive the full therapeutic benefits. (Note that when washing oily hair, shampoo should be applied before wetting the hair to help emulsify the oil.)

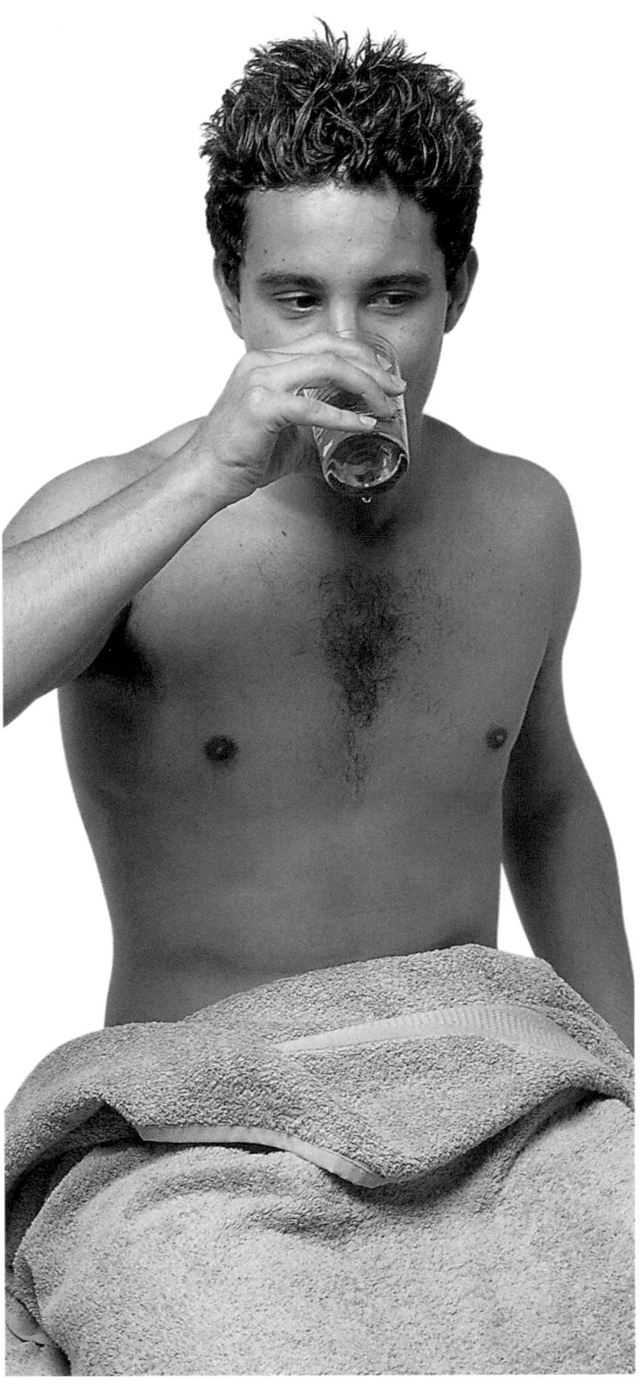

Sequence B: the lying position

ALTHOUGH INDIAN HEAD MASSAGE is usually given when the receiver is in the seated position, the lying position provides the optimum relaxation and both versions are extremely beneficial. If there is a great deal of tension in the shoulders and upper back, it is easier to tackle when the receiver is in the seated position. If, however, you wish to concentrate on the receiver's face, it is easier to do so with the receiver lying down. Try both versions to discover which suits you best.

Prepare your treatment area by placing a duvet, futon, sleeping bag or blankets on the floor. If you have a massage couch, spread a bath sheet over it. Ask the receiver to lie on his or her back and then place one or two pillows or cushions under their head and one under their knees. If you are working on the floor, make yourself more comfortable by putting a cushion or pillow under your own knees. Cover the receiver with a towel or blanket to make them feel warm and secure.

Because I have already described the Indian head massage in full for the seated position, I will now outline a shortened version for the lying position, which will probably take you about fifteen minutes. You may, of course, incorporate any of the techniques that I have detailed for the seated version.

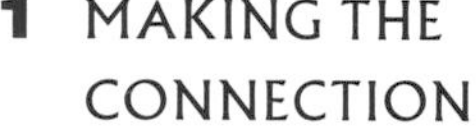

1 MAKING THE CONNECTION

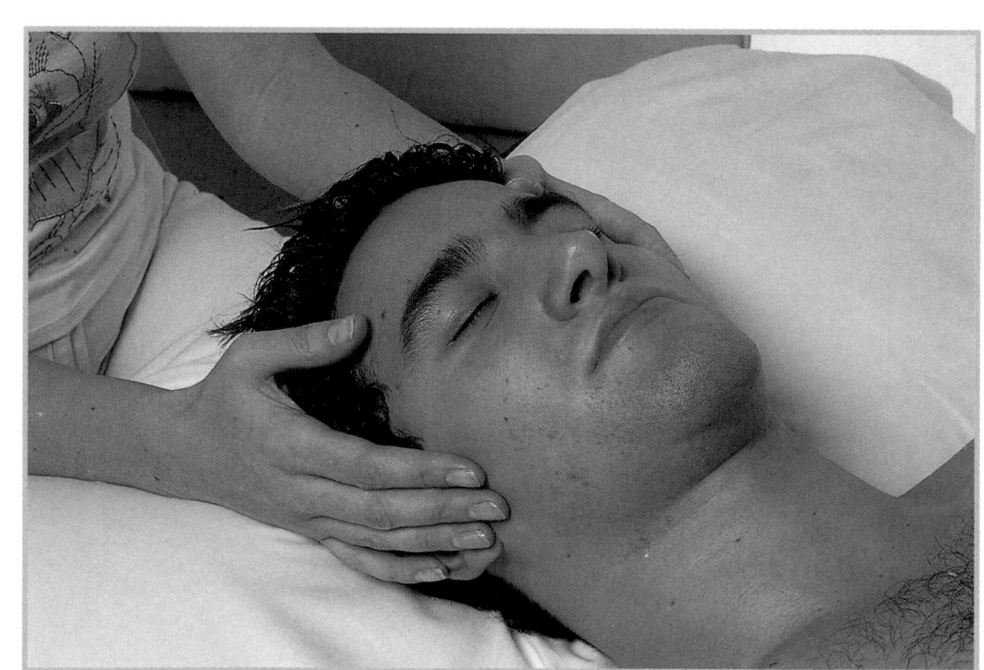

Position yourself behind the receiver. Place your hands very gently on their head and sit quietly for a minute or so until you and your partner feel completely relaxed. Notice how your partner's breathing slows and deepens as tension is released.

The upper back, shoulders and arms sequence

2 EFFLEURAGING THE BACK

Place your hands under the receiver's back, with one palm under each shoulder blade.

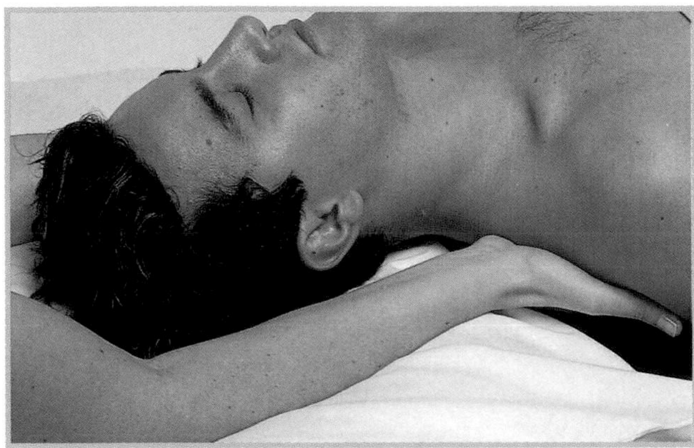

Perform large, circular movements, working outwards and using both hands simultaneously. Repeat the procedure seven times.

3 RUBBING THE UPPER BACK

Place your hand under the receiver's back, with your palms facing upwards,. Briskly rub your palms up and down until the receiver's back feels warm and as though it is glowing.

4 FRICTIONING THE BACK

i) Reach your hands as far down the receiver's back as you can manage. Place the pads of your fingers close to, but not directly on, the spine. Now make small, deep, circular movements up the receiver's back. If you find any knots or nodules of tension, either perform circular friction over them or press into, and then release, these trouble spots.

ii) For a deeper treatment, form your hands into fists and use your knuckles to perform the friction. You may also friction around each of the shoulder blades to release any knots and nodules of tension.

5 OPENING-OUT THE CHEST

Place both of your hands in the centre of the receiver's upper chest.

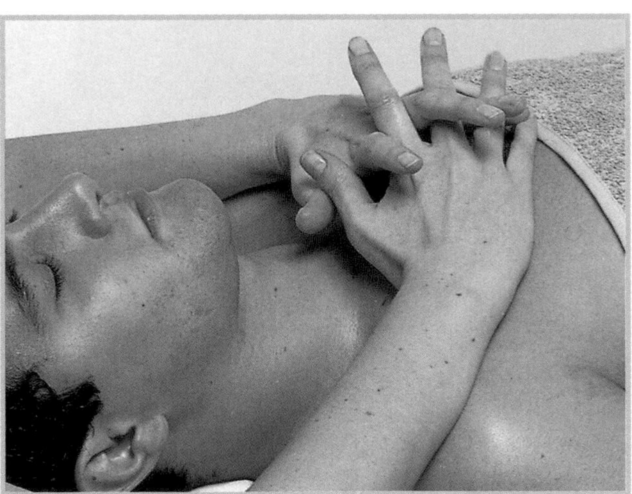

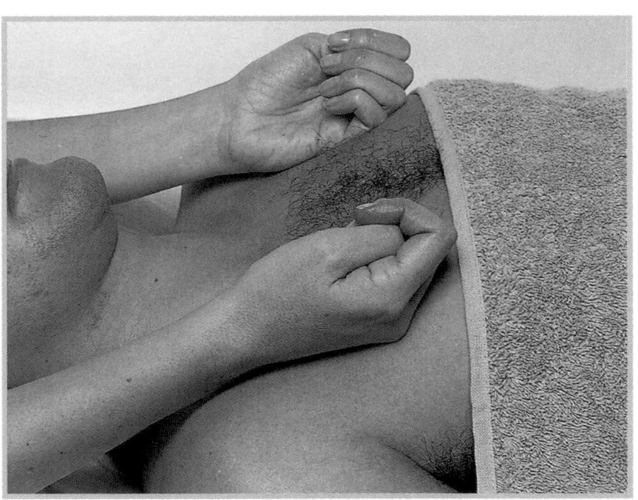

i) Now stroke outwards, towards the armpits, before allowing your hands to glide back lightly to your starting point. Repeat the procedure several times.

ii) Curl your hands into loose fists and perform gentle, circular movements over all of the upper chest area to loosen the muscles.

6 EFFLEURAGING THE SHOULDERS AND UPPER ARMS

Place your hands on each of the receiver's shoulders. Use the heels of your hands to stroke firmly across the top of the shoulders and then down the upper arms until you reach the elbows.

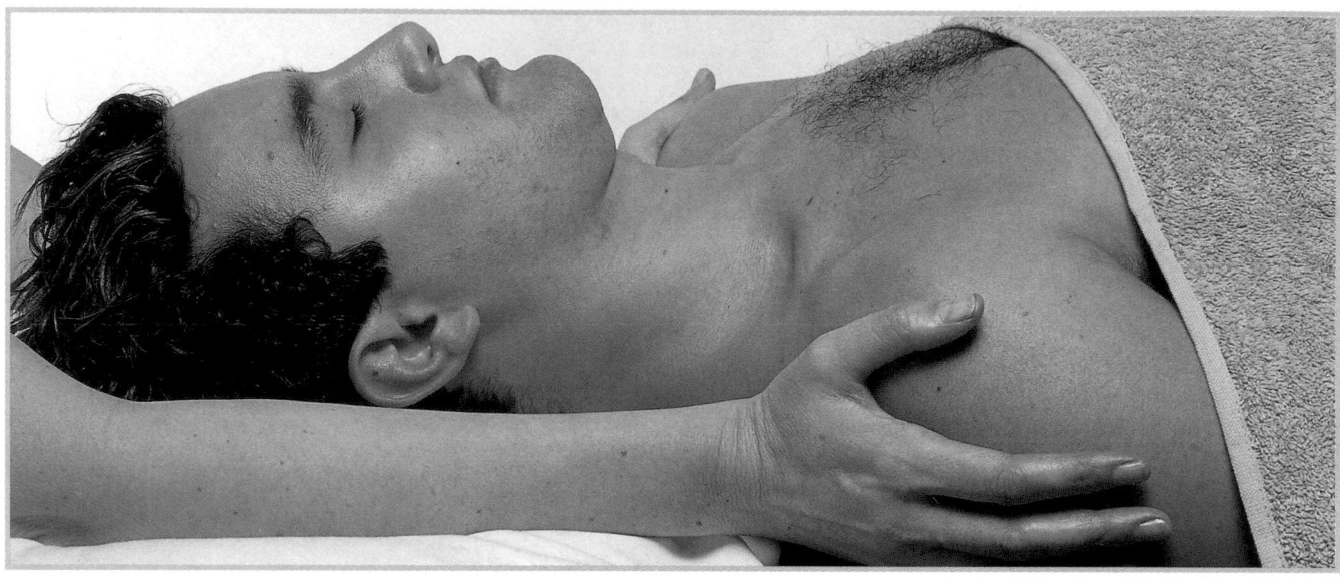

7 SQUEEZING AND WRINGING THE UPPER ARMS

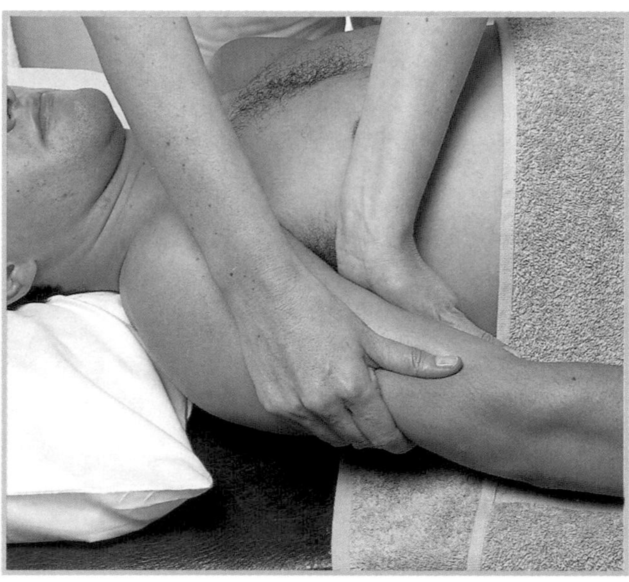

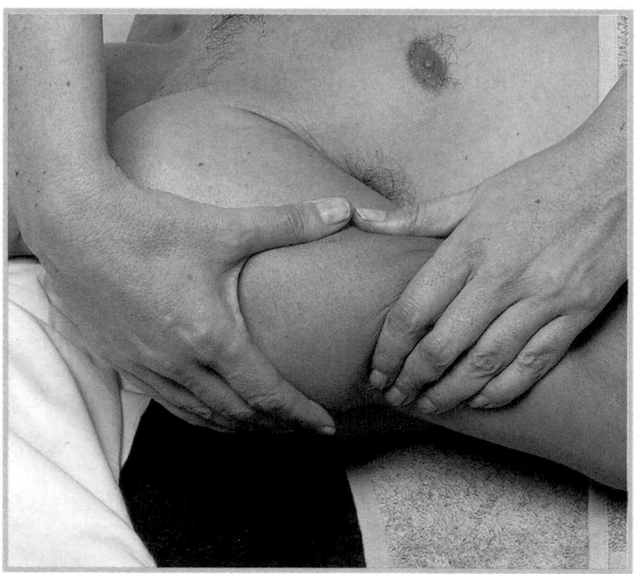

Position yourself at the receiver's side.

i) Place the palms of both of your hands around an upper arm, one on the front and one on the back. Gently squeeze and release the muscles as you work towards the elbow and then back again. Repeat the procedure several times.

ii) Still working on the same side, rhythmically wring the upper arm using alternate hands. As you do so, pick up as much muscle as you can.

Repeat the squeezing and wringing processes on the other arm.

8 KNUCKLING THE SHOULDERS

Position yourself behind the receiver. Form your hands into fists and place your knuckles on each of the receiver's shoulders.

Now perform circular movements with your knuckled fists as you work across the top of the shoulders and then back again.

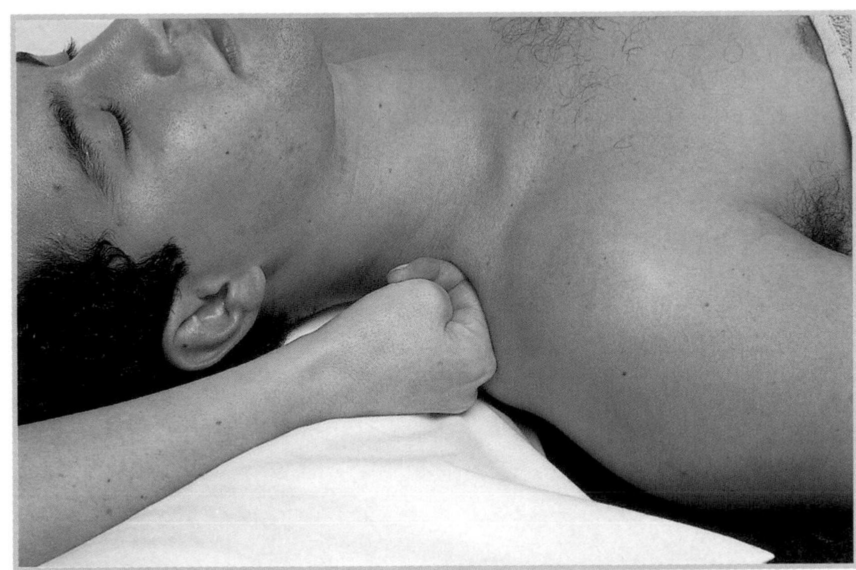

9 WRINGING THE SHOULDERS

Position yourself in front, and to the side, of your partner.

Place both hands on the shoulder opposite you, with your palms facing downwards. Now wring the muscles using alternate hands. Change sides and repeat the wringing procedure on the other shoulder.

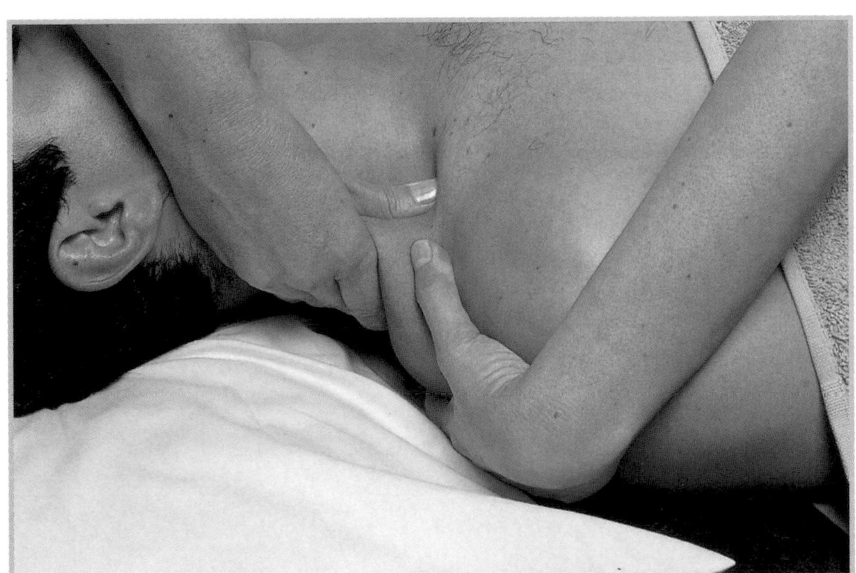

10 SHOULDER STRETCHES

Cup your hands around each of the receiver's shoulders.

Push them downwards, towards your partner's feet. Now place your hands on the front of the receiver's shoulders and gently push them downwards, towards the massage surface.

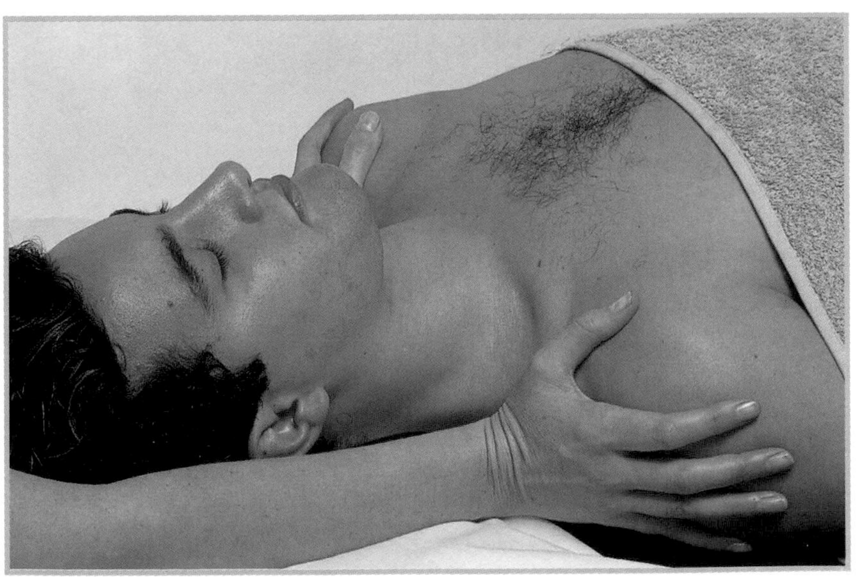

The neck sequence

1 EFFLEURAGING THE NECK

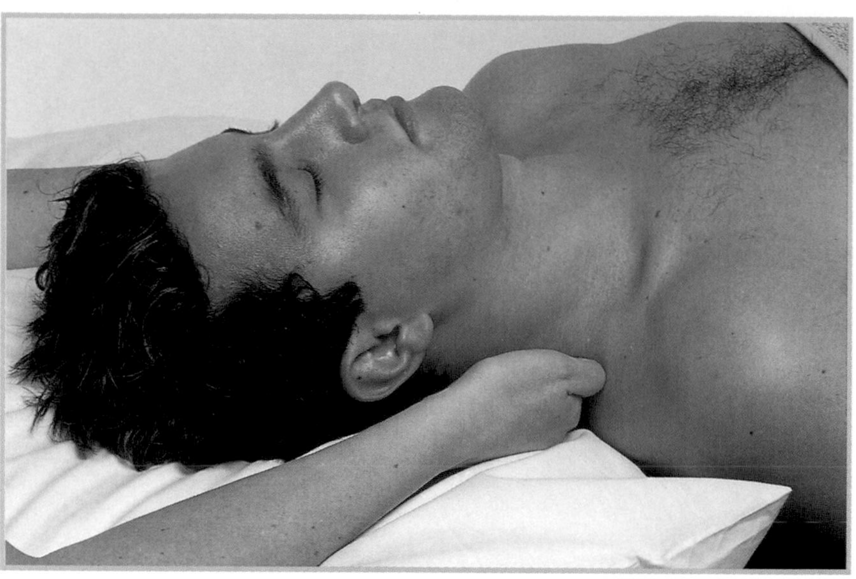

Seat yourself at the receiver's head, where you should remain for the entire neck sequence.

Place both of your hands under your partner's neck, one hand above the other. Gently pull both sides of the neck upwards, towards you. Repeat the procedure until you feel the neck relaxing and the tension dissolving.

2 FRICTIONING THE NECK

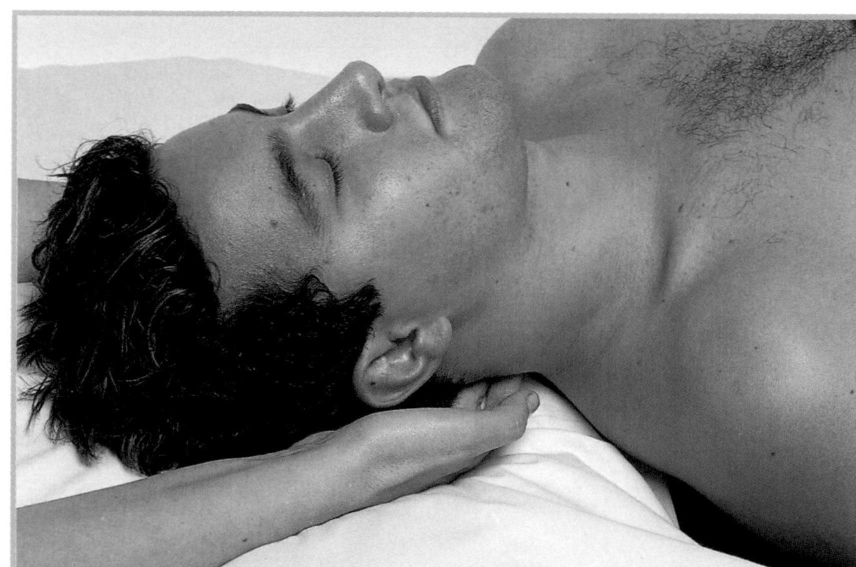

Place the fleshy pads of your fingers on the back of the receiver's neck.

Now make small, circular, outward-pointing movements as you work from the base of the neck up towards the base of the skull. The neck is a delicate area, so apply only very gentle pressure.

3 SIDE STROKING THE NECK

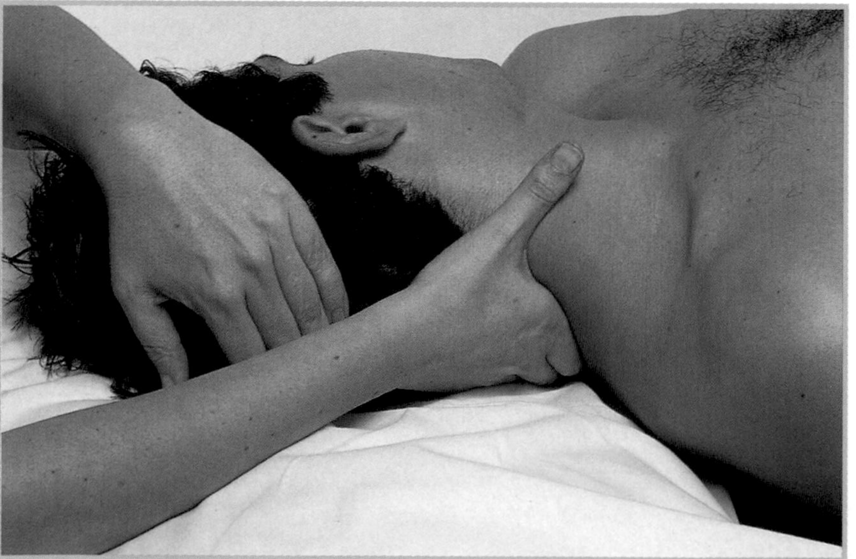

Gently turn the receiver's head to one side and place one hand at the back of their head to provide support.

Use your other hand to stroke down the side of the neck, working from the base of the skull towards the shoulder.

4 FRICTIONING THE SIDE OF THE NECK

Keep the neck in the same position, and support the receiver's head with one hand.

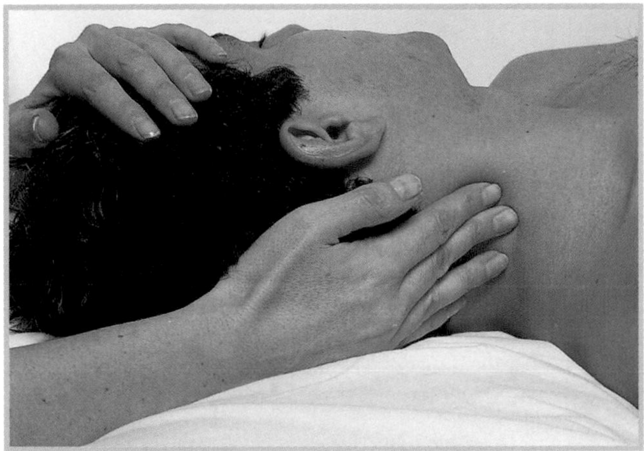

Use the fingertips of your other hand to perform gentle, circular, outward-pointing movements down the side of the neck. Remember not to apply too much pressure.

6 FRICTIONING UNDER THE BASE OF THE SKULL

Supporting the reciever's head, position the pads of your fingers at the base of the receiver's skull (occiput).

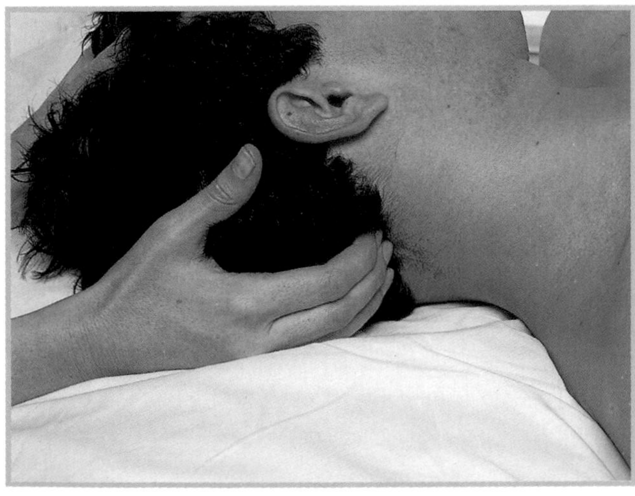

Now perform gentle, circular movements all along the skull.

5 SQUEEZING THE SIDE OF THE NECK

Still keeping the neck in the same position, continue to support the receiver's head with one hand.

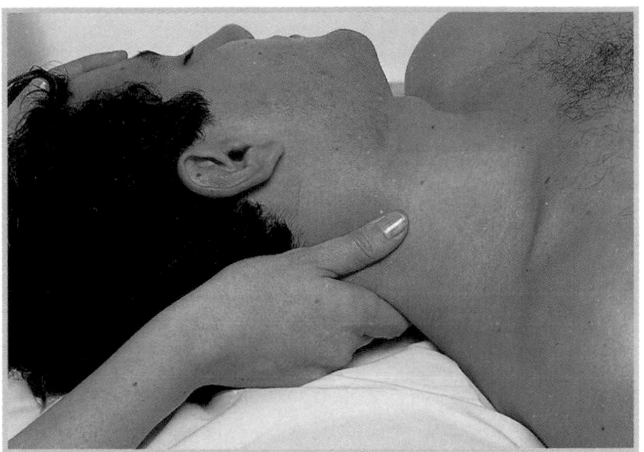

Place your other hand, with the palm facing downwards, on the side of the neck so that your thumb and fingers form a 'V' shape. Gently squeeze and release the neck muscles.

Switch to the other side of the neck and repeat steps 3, 4 and 5.

7 HOLDING THE NECK

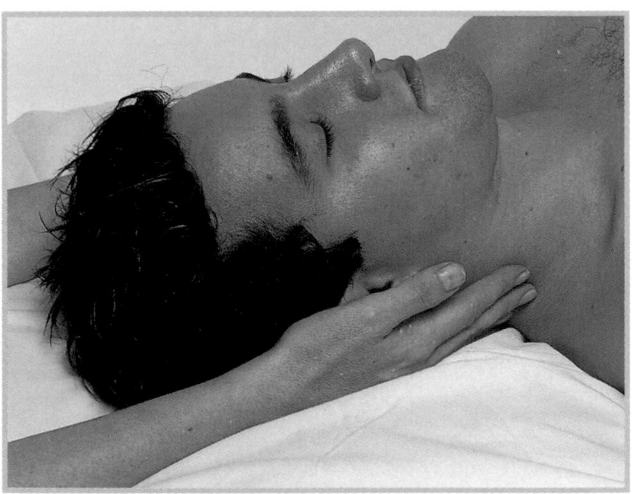

Place your hands very lightly on the receiver's neck and rest them there for thirty seconds or more. Feel how warm and relaxed the neck has become.

The scalp and facial sequence

1 CONNECTING WITH THE RECEIVER

Rest your hands, with the palms facing downwards, on the receiver's forehead, so gently that you're hardly touching it.

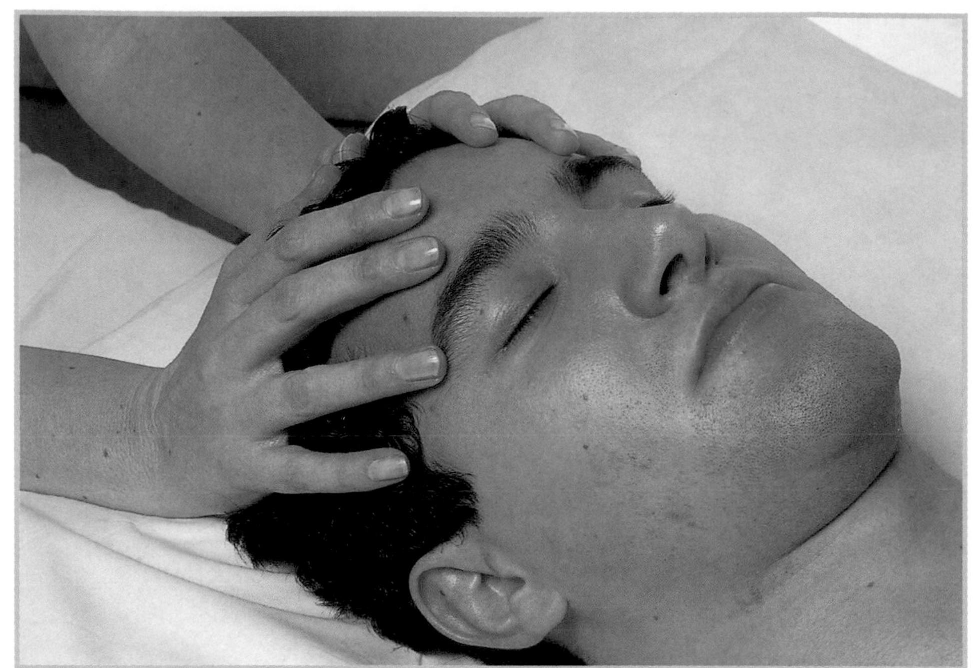

2 STROKING THE FACE

i) First place the palms of your hands on the receiver's forehead, with your fingers interlocking.

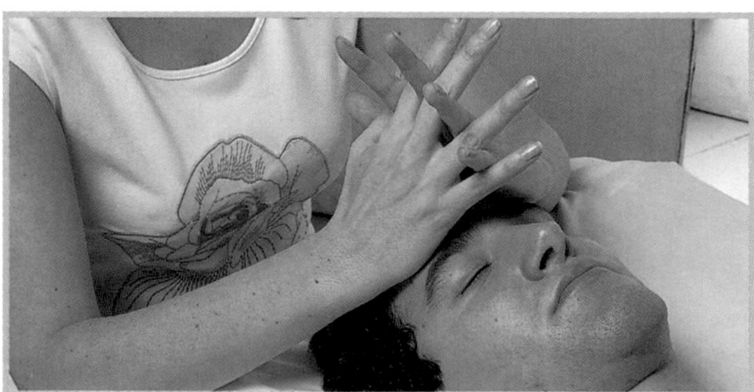

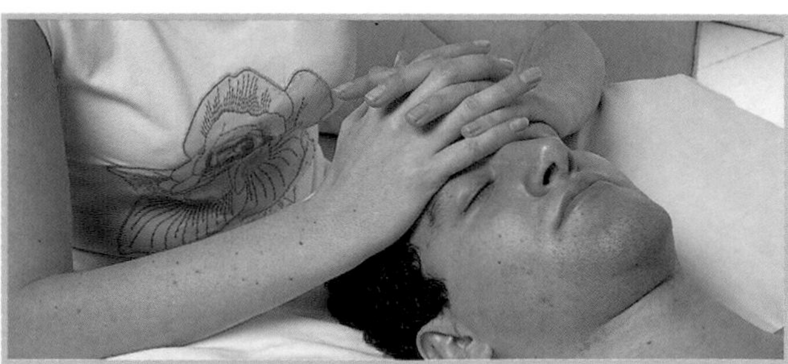

ii) Gently draw your fingers apart as you start stroking outwards, across the forehead. Allow your hands to glide back to your starting position before repeating the movement several times.

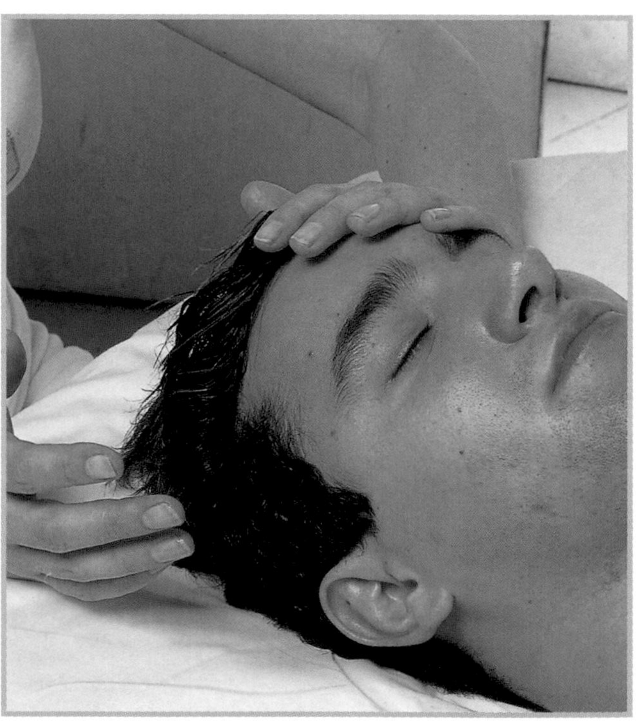

iii) Alternatively, place one hand across the centre of the receiver's forehead. Stroke this hand outwards, towards the temple, and as it completes the movement, stroke your other hand across the receiver's forehead.

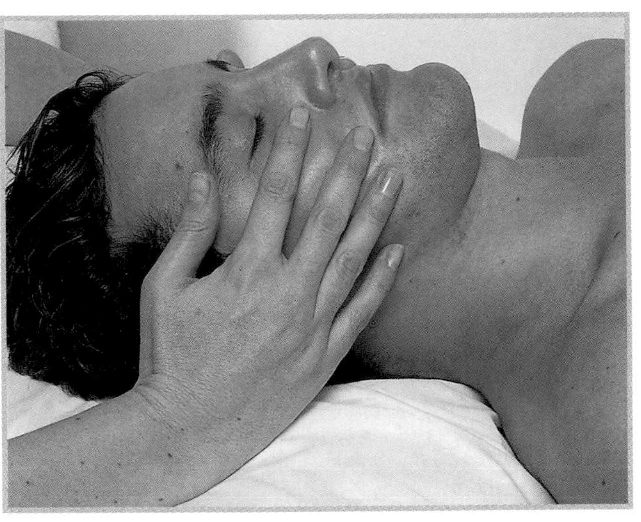

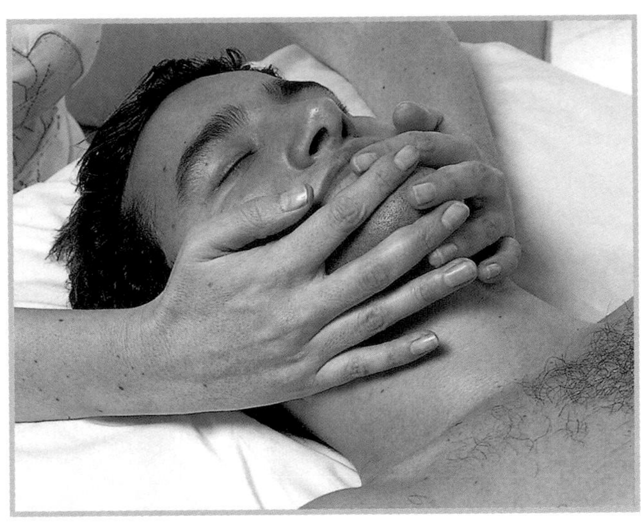

iv) Place one hand on each of the receiver's cheeks and then stroke them outwards.

v) Place your hands in the centre of the receiver's chin and again stroke them outwards. If you wish, you may continue the movement down the neck and towards the shoulders.

3 PRESSING AND RELEASING THE FACIAL PRESSURE POINTS

First place the pads of your thumbs in the centre of the receiver's forehead, just below the hairline.

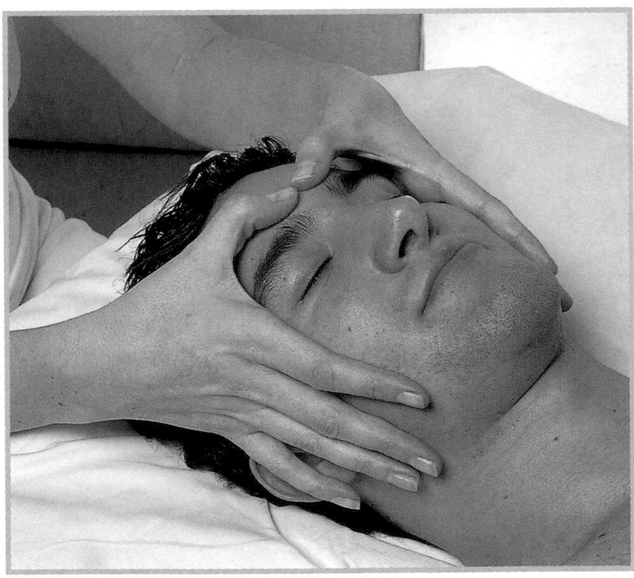

i) Press your thumbs into the receiver's skin and then release them. Now move your thumbs slightly outwards and press and release again. Continue working outwards in a horizontal row.

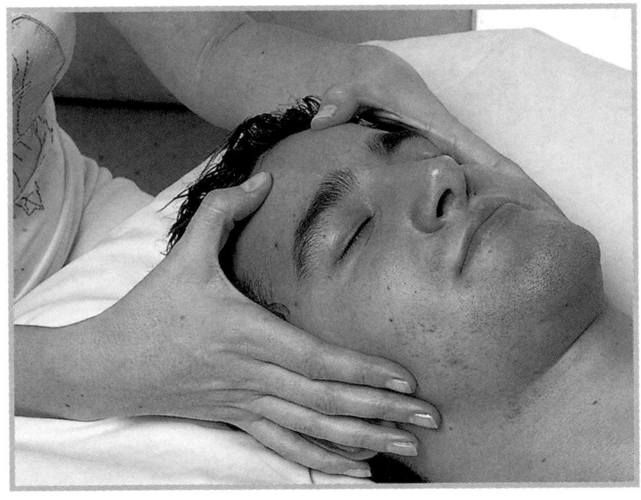

ii) After completing the first row, bring your thumbs back to the centre of the forehead, but place them slightly lower down. Repeat another row of pressure points. Continue pressing and releasing in horizontal rows until you reach the top of the receiver's eyebrows.

iii) Place the pads of your thumbs next to the receiver's nose, just below the eyes. Gently pressing and releasing, work outwards across the cheeks, following the line of the cheekbones. Continue working in horizontal strips as you did for the forehead until you reach the receiver's mouth.

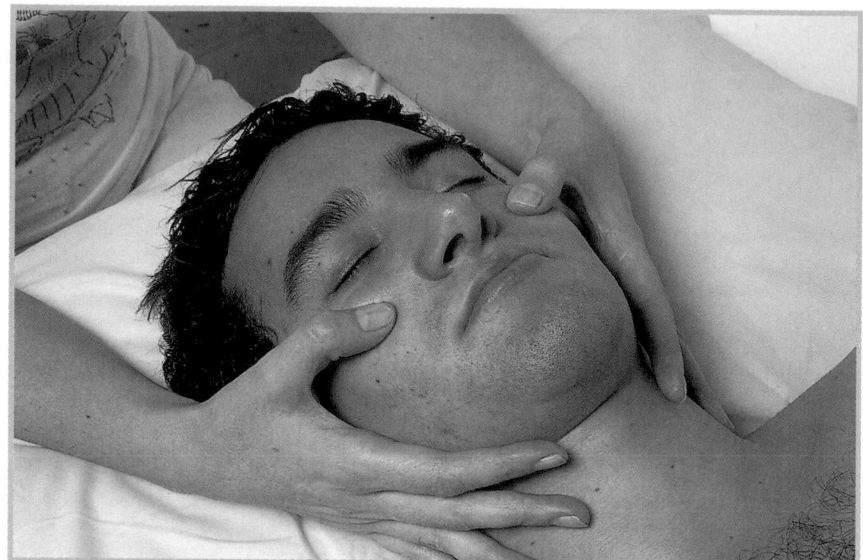

iv) Repeat the pressing-and-releasing procedure over the receiver's chin area.

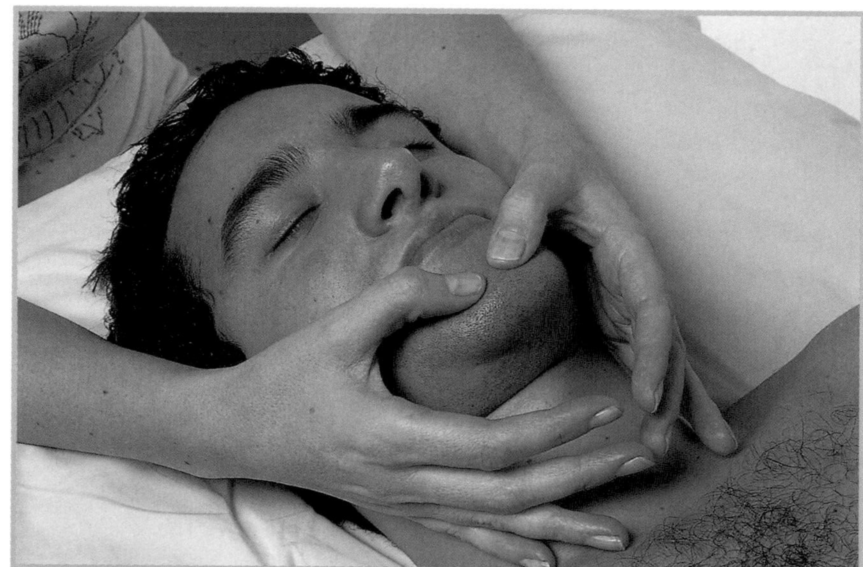

4 RELEASING JAW TENSION

Lightly hook your fingertips around the receiver's jawbone. Then perform gentle, circular friction movements, working from the centre of the jaw towards the ears. Place your thumb on the front of the receiver's chin, and your index finger underneath it, and then gently squeeze and release the jaw.

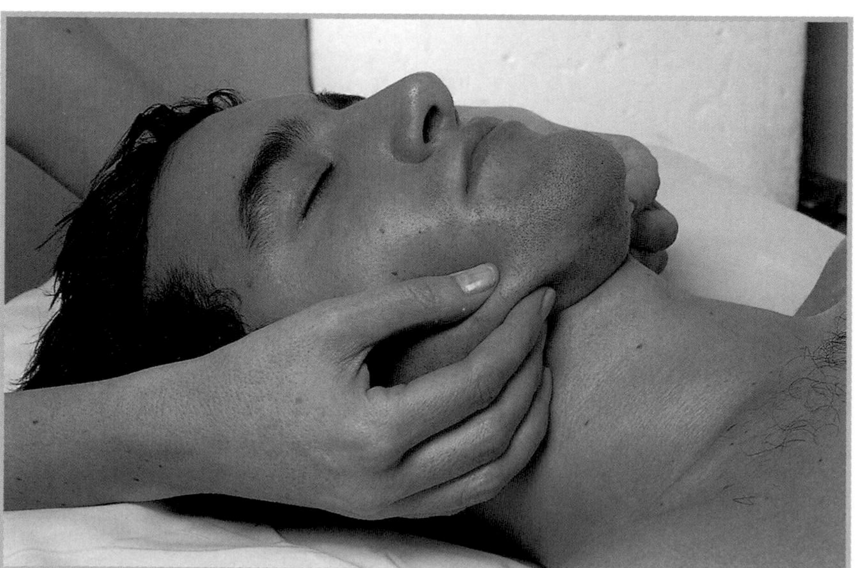

5 SQUEEZING THE EYEBROWS

Using your thumb and index finger, gently squeeze the receiver's eyebrows, working from the inner to the outer edge.

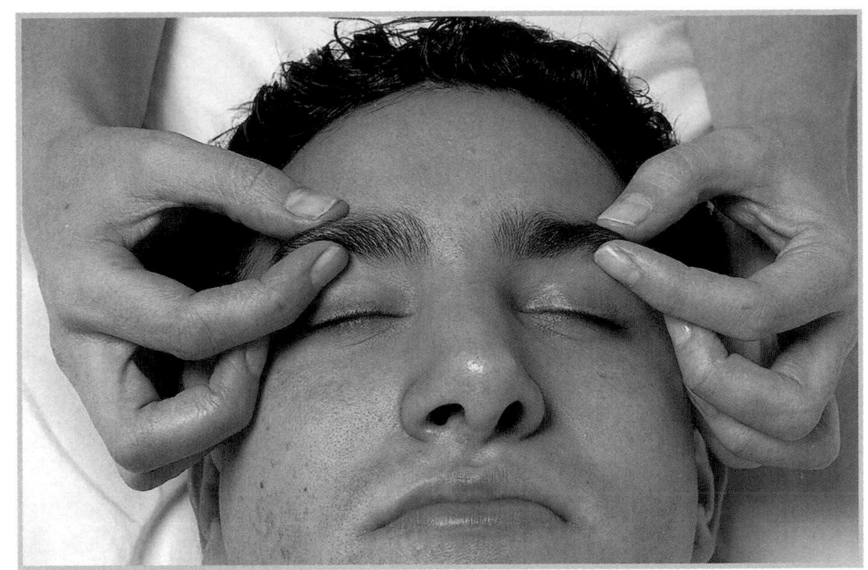

6 MASSAGING THE EARS

Place the thumbs and forefingers of both hands around each of the receiver's earlobes. Massage over all of the ears before slowly and gently stretching them.

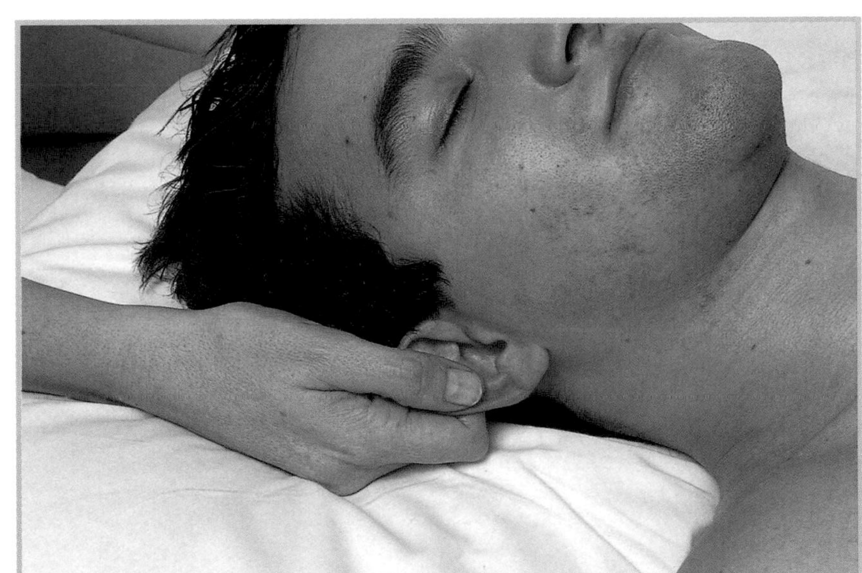

7 CIRCLING THE FACE

Place the four fingers of each of your hands just below the receiver's hairline, with your fingers pointing downwards.

Now perform small, circular movements with your fingertips as you work down the receiver's forehead to their chin and jaw.

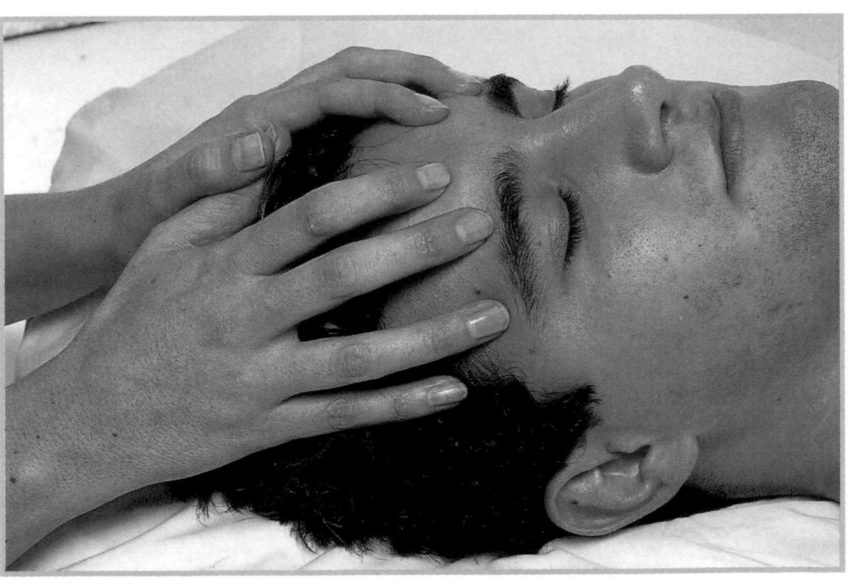

8 FACIAL TAPPING

Using the pads of your fingers, lightly tap over all of the receiver's face and under their chin.

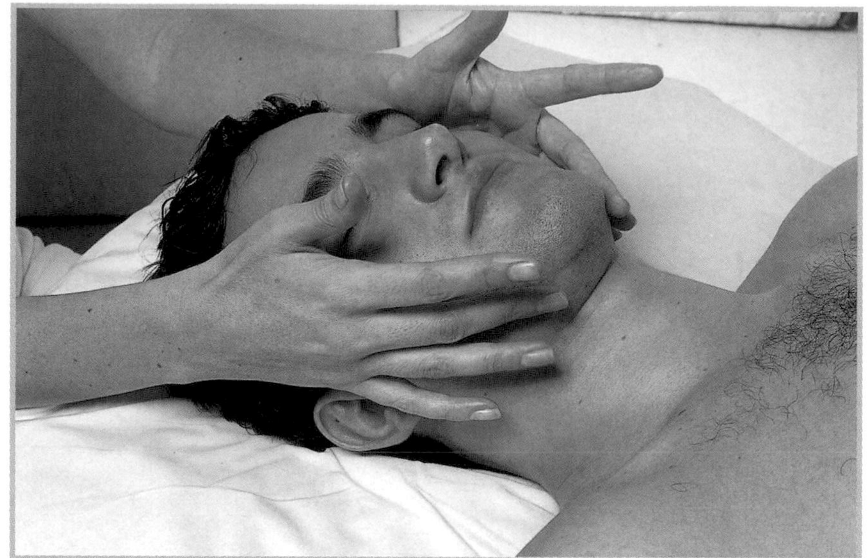

9 DISSOLVING EYE TENSION

Ask your partner to close their eyes. Then gently place your palms over their eyes and hold them there for about thirty seconds.

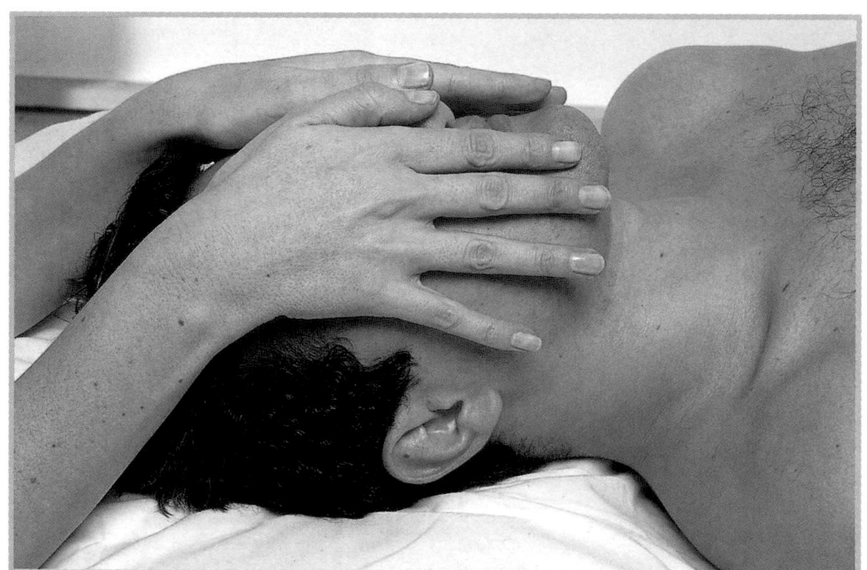

10 RUBBING THE SCALP

Turn the receiver's head slightly to one side and gently rest one hand on their forehead.

Place the palm of your other hand on the receiver's head and rub it briskly over all of the scalp. Turn the receiver's head slightly to the other side and continue rubbing briskly until you have covered the entire scalp.

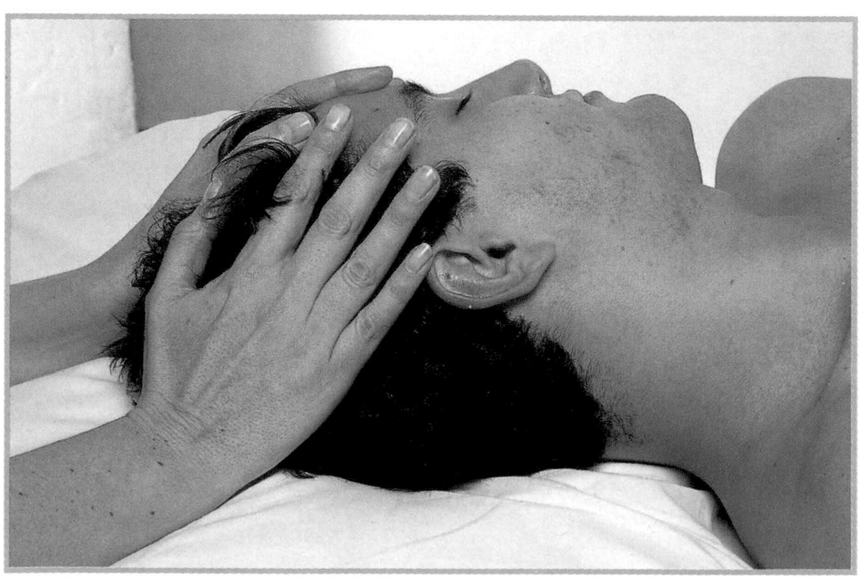

11 WHOLE HAND FRICTIONING

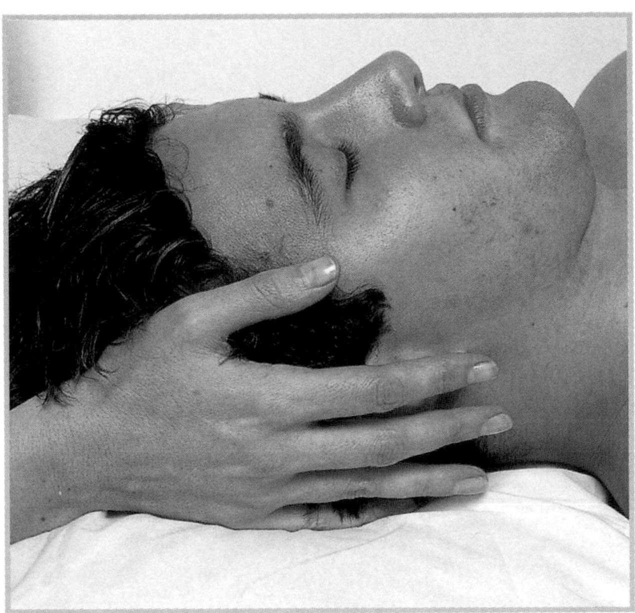

Place the palms of your hands on either side of the receiver's head. Now massage the whole of the head using a circular motion.

12 FINGER PAD FRICTIONING ('SHAMPOOING')

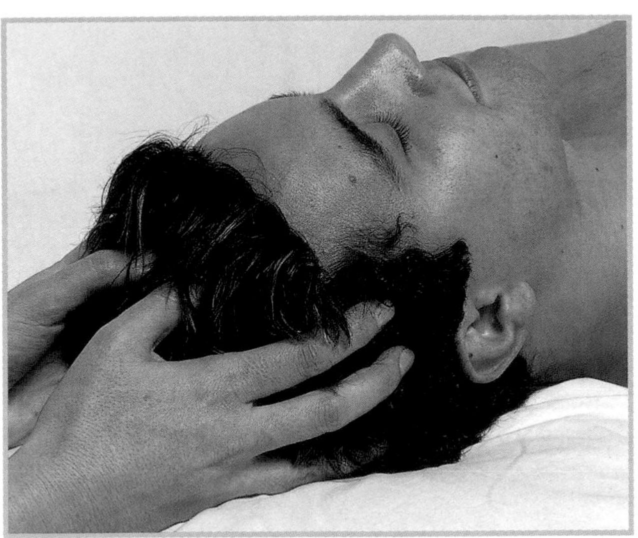

Place the fleshy pads of your fingers and thumbs on top of the receiver's head, making sure that they are well spread out. Using fairly firm pressure, perform circular movements over all of the scalp.

13 RUFFLING THE HAIR

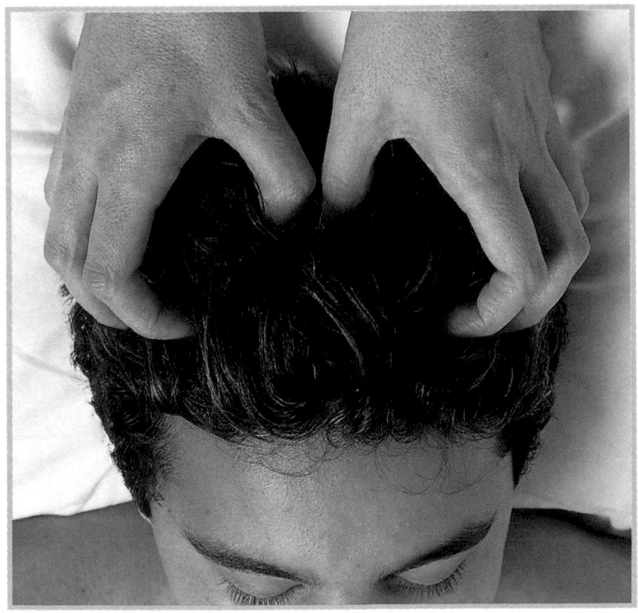

Form a claw-like shape with your hands and rest them on the receiver's scalp. Keeping your wrists loose and relaxed, gently ruffle your partner's hair.

14 'COMBING' OR TUGGING THE HAIR

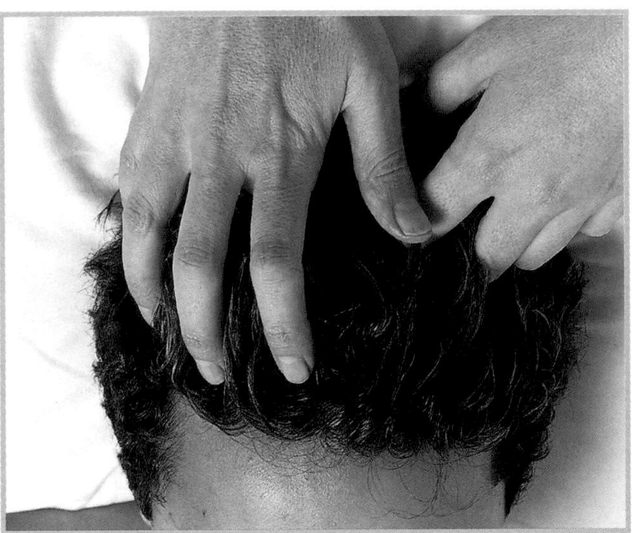

Gently 'comb' through the receiver's hair with all of the fingers of one hand, closely followed by the fingers of the other. Then turn your hands over so that the palms are facing upwards. Gather up small handfuls of hair and slowly and gently tug at it.

15 TABLA PLAYING ON THE SCALP

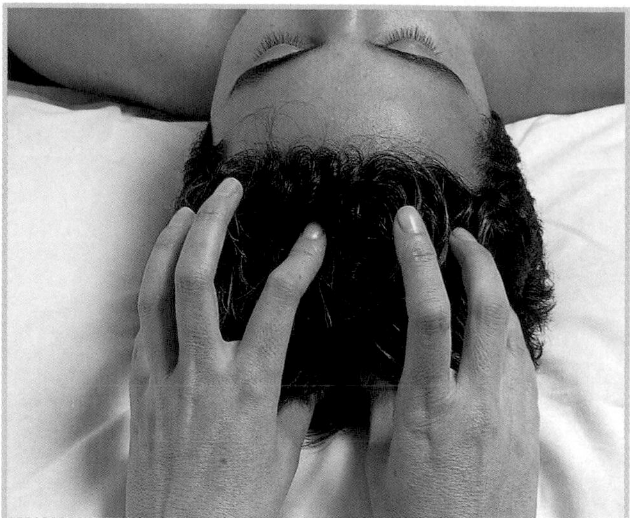

Using your fingertips, lightly tap (or drum) over all of the receiver's scalp. You may use either one or two fingertips or all of them.

16 THE FINAL TOUCH

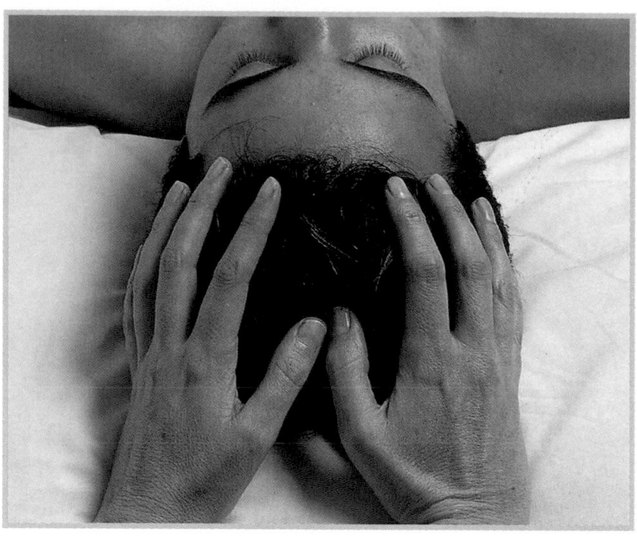

Place your hands on the receiver's head and rest them there for about thirty seconds before gradually releasing them.

The chakrabalancing sequence

Refer to Chapter 4 for detailed explanations of the chakras, as well as of chakra balancing (see also pages 55 to 56 and 80 to 81.

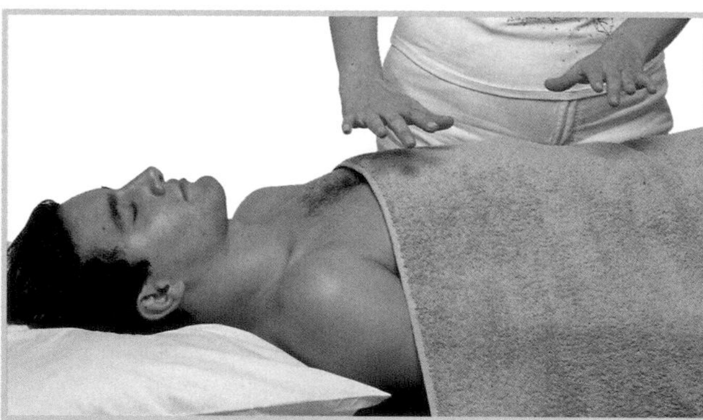

Position yourself at your partner's side. Ensure that you feel grounded by visualising imaginary roots stretching from your feet deep into the centre of the earth. Let your hands hover over the front of the receiver's body, level with the base of the spine. As you slowly allow your hands to glide up the body, visualise the following colours:

- base chakra: clear, deep red;
- sacral chakra: vibrant orange;
- solar plexus chakra: radiant gold;
- heart chakra: flower pink;
- throat chakra: clear blue;
- brow chakra: indigo;
- crown chakra: violet.

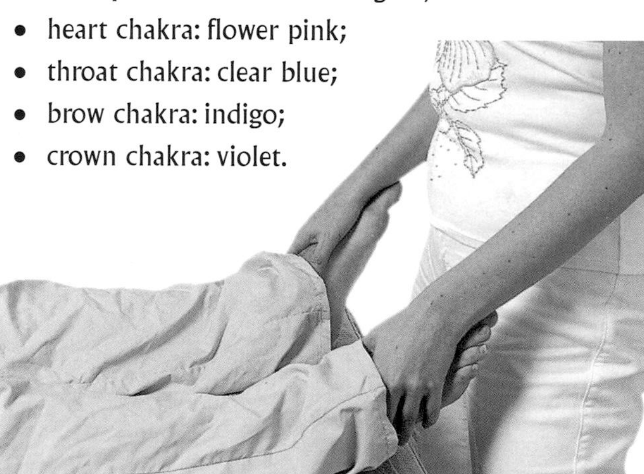

Allow the receiver slowly to rouse him- or herself from their deep state of relaxation. Then move to their feet and gently rub them to bring them back to earth. When the receiver has opened his or her eyes, offer them a glass of water.

Reactions to an Indian head massage

FOLLOWING AN INDIAN HEAD MASSAGE, several reactions may occur. This is an excellent, very positive, sign that the treatment has really worked because the reactions indicate that body is ridding itself of toxins, both mental and physical.

The reactions may include:

- an excellent night's sleep;
- improved concentration and clarity of thought;
- relief from stress and tension;
- varying degrees of tiredness, followed by a surge in energy levels;
- increased vitality;
- feelings of peace and harmony;
- a slight aching and soreness in the muscles, particularly those that needed extra work due to the build-up of knots of tension;
- a heightened emotional state, during which the receiver may be tearful or giggly;
- an increased frequency of bowel movements and urination as toxins are released;
- increased perspiration and mucus production;
- a slight, temporary, skin rash.

Aftercare

In order to derive the maximum benefit from an Indian head massage, the receiver should follow these guidelines.

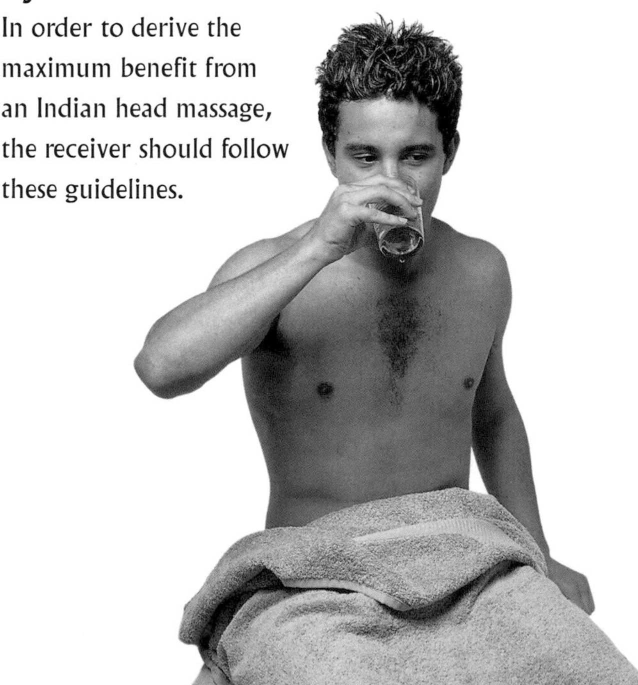

INCREASE YOUR WATER INTAKE

Increasing your water intake will greatly assist and accelerate the detoxification process. Water not only detoxifies the body and boosts energy levels, but also enables us to fight off infections and to look years younger. Drinking eight glasses a day is recommended to improve your health and well-being.

CUT DOWN YOUR CAFFEINE AND ALCOHOL INTAKES

Tea, coffee and other caffeinated drinks, as well as alcohol, put great strain on the systems of the body and overstimulate the kidneys in particular. Along with water, try drinking herbal teas or freshly prepared fruit or vegetable juices instead.

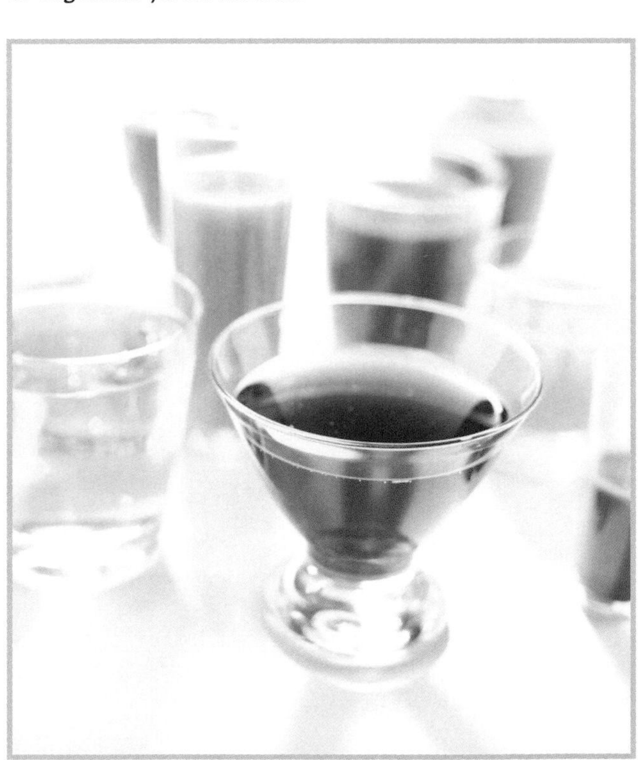

AVOID EATING HEAVY MEALS

Your diet should be light to enable your body to use its energy for healing rather than digestion. Fruits, vegetables and salads should form a major part of a well-balanced diet. Food packed with preservatives and colourings should be avoided, as well as too much fat and sugar, all of which can cause health problems.

STOP SMOKING

We are all aware of the dangers of smoking and of the diseases that it can cause, so why not derive your relaxation from an Indian head massage rather than a packet of cigarettes?

TAKE REGULAR EXERCISE

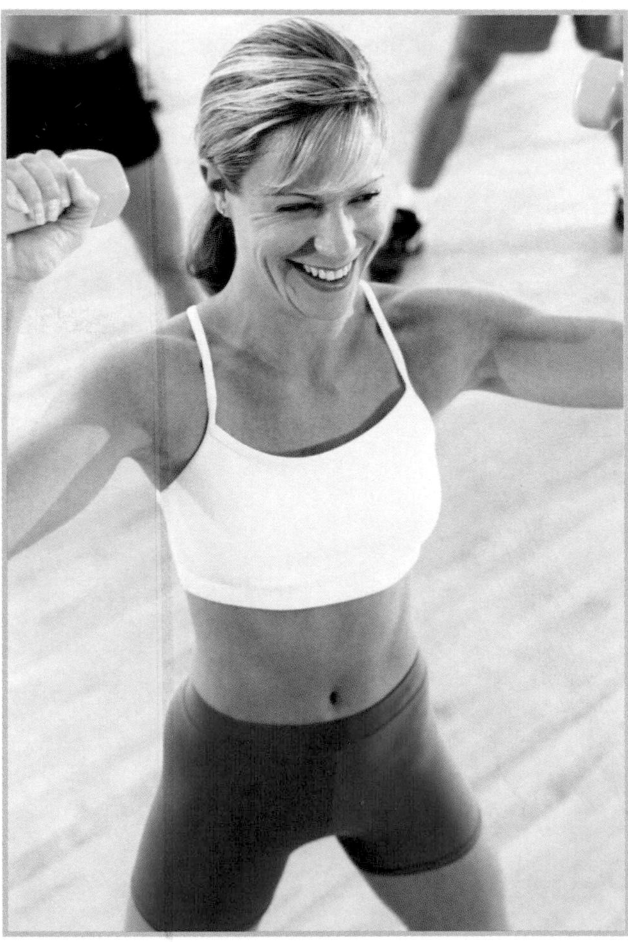

Taking regular exercise will increase your vitality, improve your circulation, tone your muscles and relieve any tension. All in all, exercise is an excellent preventative medicine.

GET ENOUGH SLEEP

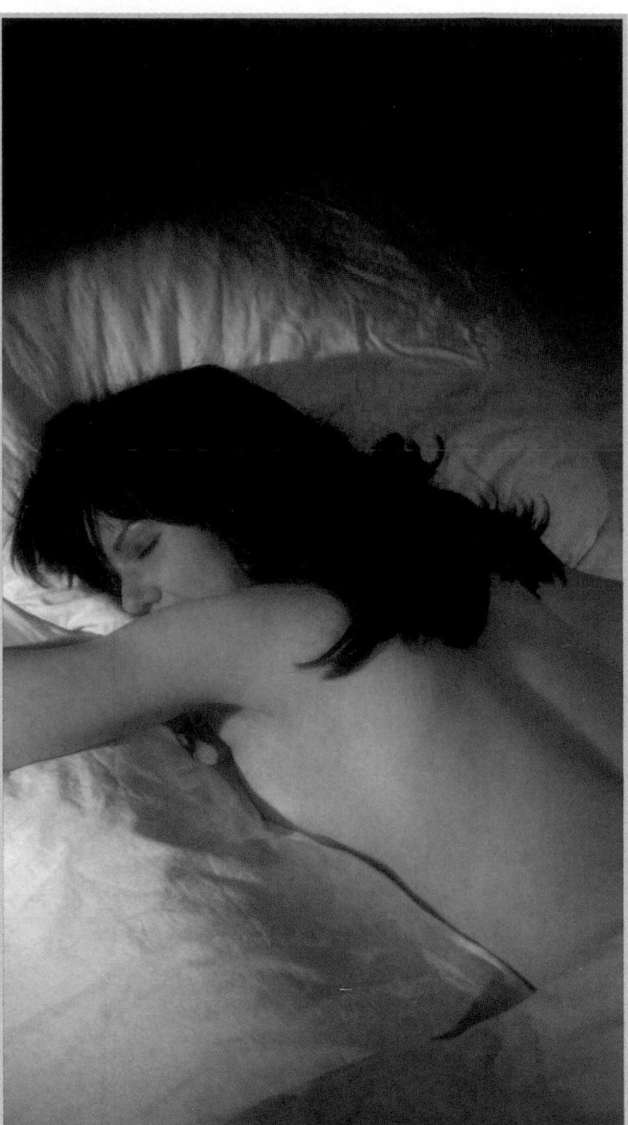

Sleep is essential for healing. Having a good night's sleep will enable you to feel refreshed and ready to face the challenges of the day when you wake up. Lack of sleep, on the other hand, causes irritability and sluggishness.

RELAX

Reorganise your life so that you have plenty of time to enjoy some rest and relaxation, which will in turn enable you to handle the stresses and strains of life more easily. Some ideas include enjoying a massage, listening to some relaxation music, taking an aromatherapy bath, going for a walk in the fresh air and having a good laugh with your friends and family.

Self Massage

IT IS IMPORTANT THAT YOU take care of yourself, as well as of others. Although self-massage is obviously not as pleasurable as receiving a treatment given by someone else, it is still an excellent way of improving the health of your hair and skin and of keeping them in tiptop condition.

This simple self-massage routine enables you to work on your neck, shoulders, scalp and face. It can be performed as often as you wish and should ideally be incorporated into your daily routine to soothe away the day's stress andtension. The complete massage will take only about ten to fifteen minutes, so you should be able to treat yourself at least once a week to boost your energy levels and to keep stress at bay.

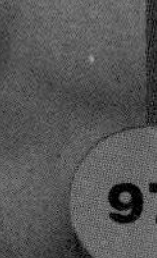

Self Massage

ALTHOUGH IT IS NOT ESSENTIAL THAT YOU USE OIL, if you do, it will help to make your hair strong, shiny and lustrous and will moisturise and balance your skin. Choose a carrier oil or, even better, a blend of oils, that is suitable for your hair and skin type (see Chapter 2).

Prepare your surroundings so that you create a peaceful, healing space in which you can relax. Unplug the phone, warm the room, soften the lighting, burn some essential oils and play some relaxation music. Make yourself comfortable by sitting either on a chair, with both of your feet on the ground, or on a few cushions spread over the floor. Ensure that you have a warm towel or two to hand in case you feel cold during the treatment.

Sit with your back held straight to allow the healing energies to flow freely. Lightly close your eyes and feel the tension melting away as you take a few deep breaths. Breathe in peace and breathe out negativity. Feel your shoulders relaxing, the tightness in your neck muscles dissolving and your facial muscles softening.

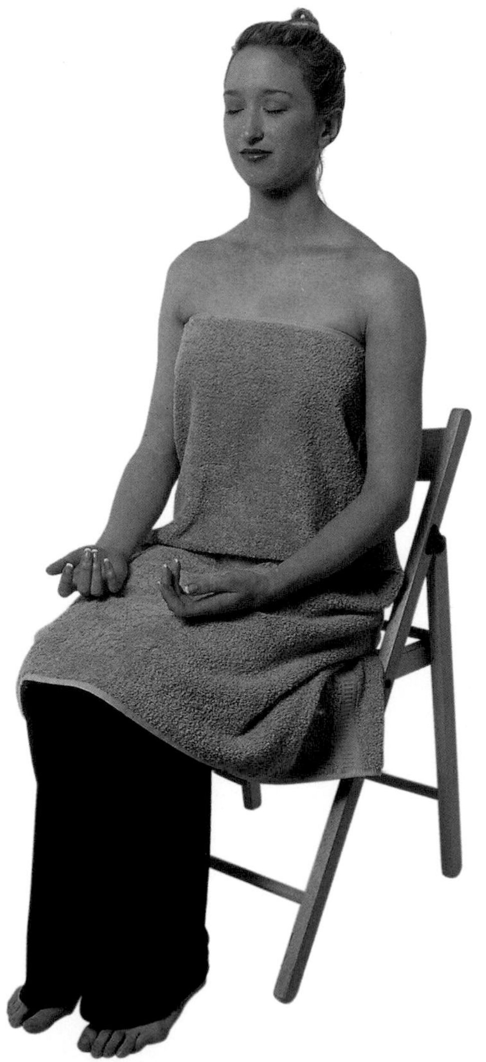

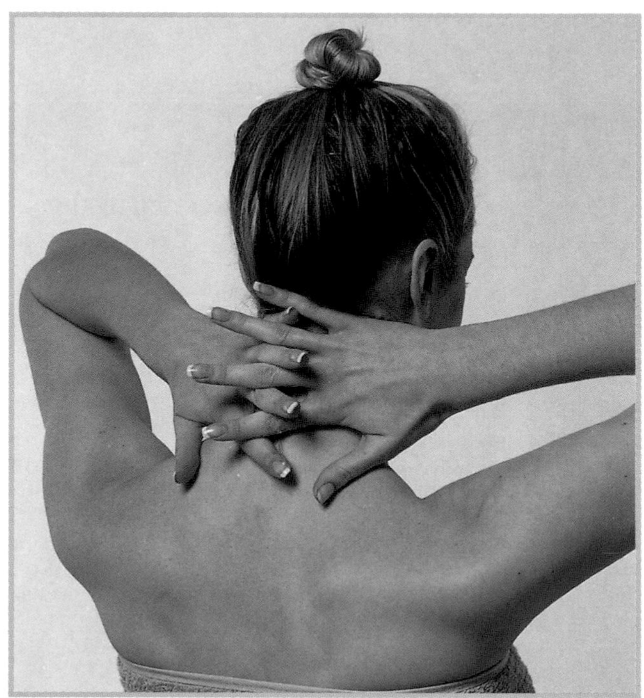

The neck and shoulders sequence

1 EFFLEURAGING YOUR NECK

Place both of your hands at the back of your neck, with your fingers lightly clasped together.

Gently pull your hands apart as you stroke the back of your neck. Repeat the procedure several times. Starting in the same position, but with your fingers slightly separated so that they are resting on either side of your spine, use your fingertips to perform circular, outward-moving effleurages over the back of your neck.

2 EFFLEURAGING ONE SIDE OF YOUR NECK

Turn your head slightly to one side and place the palm of one hand on the opposite side of your neck.

Firmly stroke down that side of your neck, bringing the palm of your hand towards the front of your neck. Repeat the procedure several times to relax your muscles thoroughly. (below)

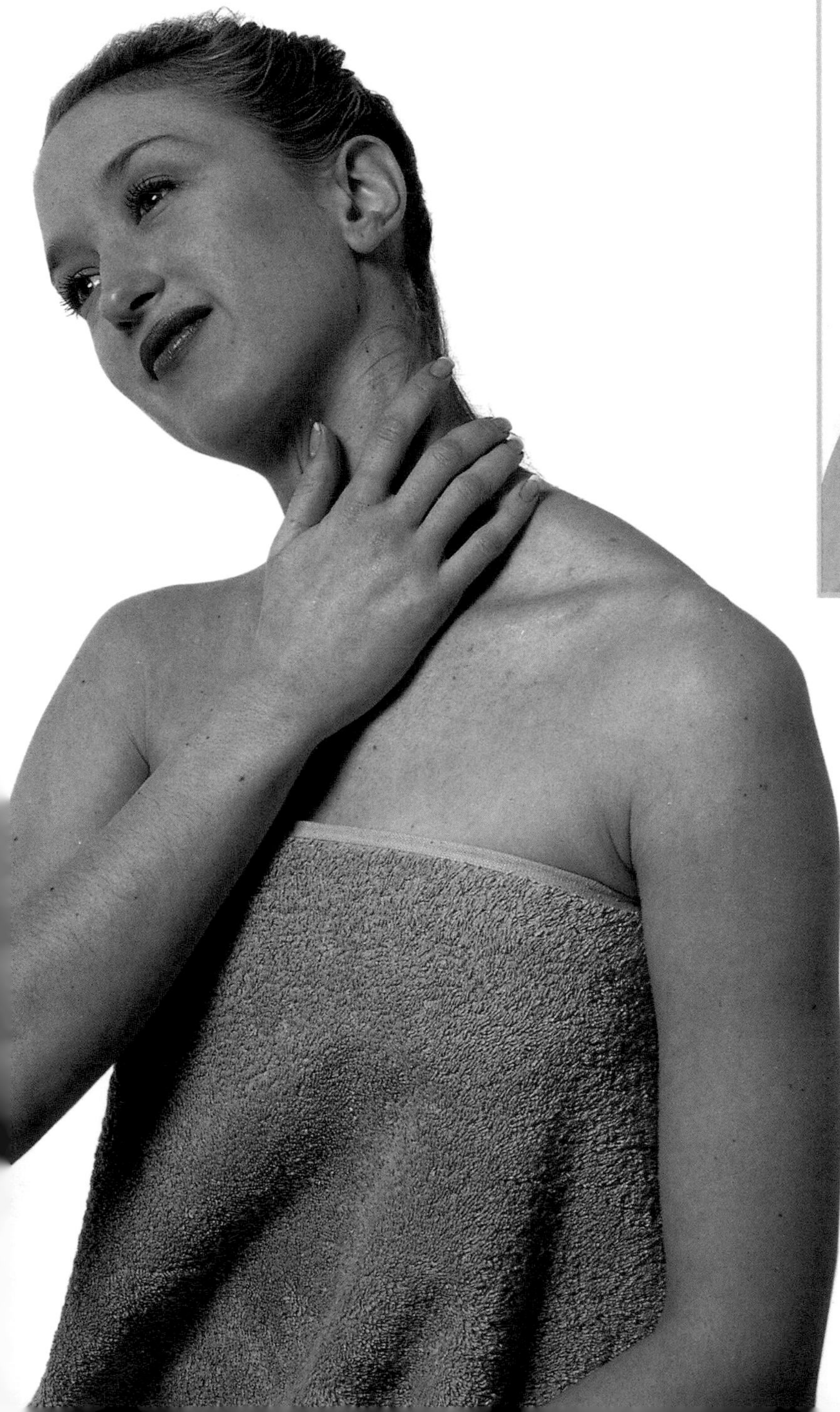

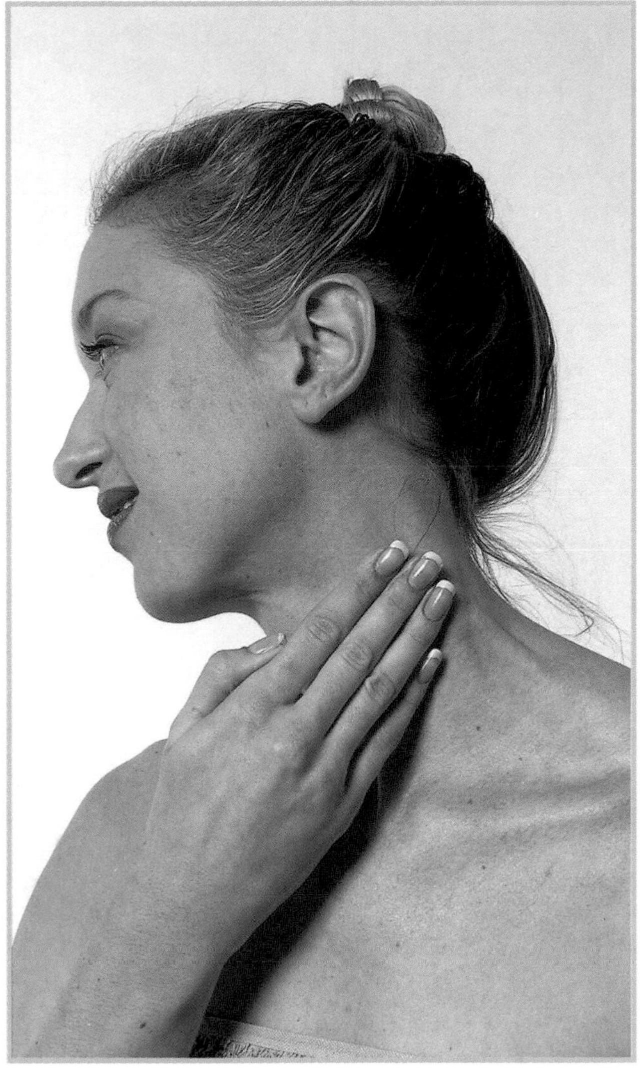

3 FRICTIONING ONE SIDE OF YOUR NECK

Still with your head turned slightly to one side, place your hand, with your palm facing downwards, at the base of your skull on the opposite side of your neck.

Use the fleshy pads of your fingertips to massage your neck gently, using a circular action as you work from the base of your skull all the way down the side of your neck. (above)

Now tilt your head to the other side, change hands and repeat steps 2 and 3 on the other side of your neck.

4 SQUEEZING YOUR SHOULDERS

Place the palm of one hand on the opposite shoulder.

Gently, but firmly, pick up and squeeze the shoulder muscles until you feel the tightness loosen. Pick up as much flesh as possible. If you find any knots of tension, perform deep, circular movements on these areas with your fingertips. Repeat the procedure on your other shoulder.

5 FRICTIONING THE BASE OF YOUR SKULL

Let your head relax by drooping forwards as far as is comfortable and then position both of your thumbs at the centre of the base of your skull (occiput).

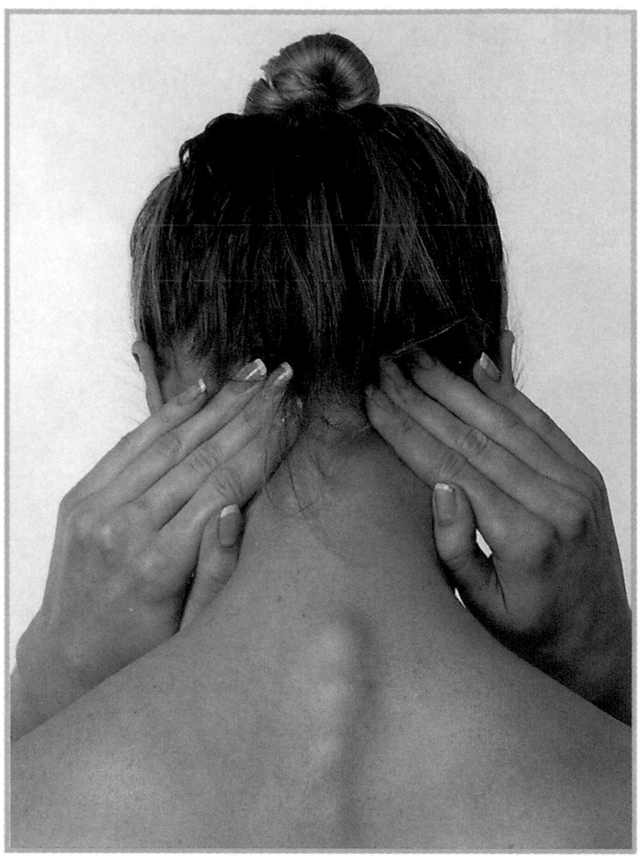

Perform small, circular, outward-moving frictions, working from the centre of your skull along its bony ridge until you reach your ears. Apply fairly light pressure to begin with, then gradually increase the pressure as far as is comfortable. Work along the base of your scalp three times. To apply lighter pressure, use the pads of your fingers. (above)

6 STROKING YOUR NECK AND SHOULDERS

To complete the neck and shoulders sequence, place each hand on either side of the top of your neck.

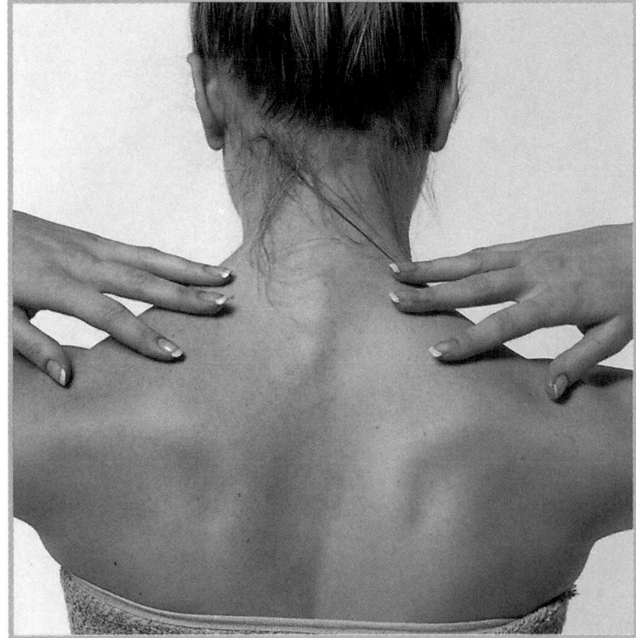

Working very slowly, stroke both hands down the back and sides of your neck and then down your shoulders.

The scalp and face sequence

1 FRICTIONING YOUR SCALP

Place both of your hands, with your palms facing downwards and your fingers interlocking slightly, on top of your head.

Use the heels of your hands to perform large, circular friction over all of your scalp. (below)

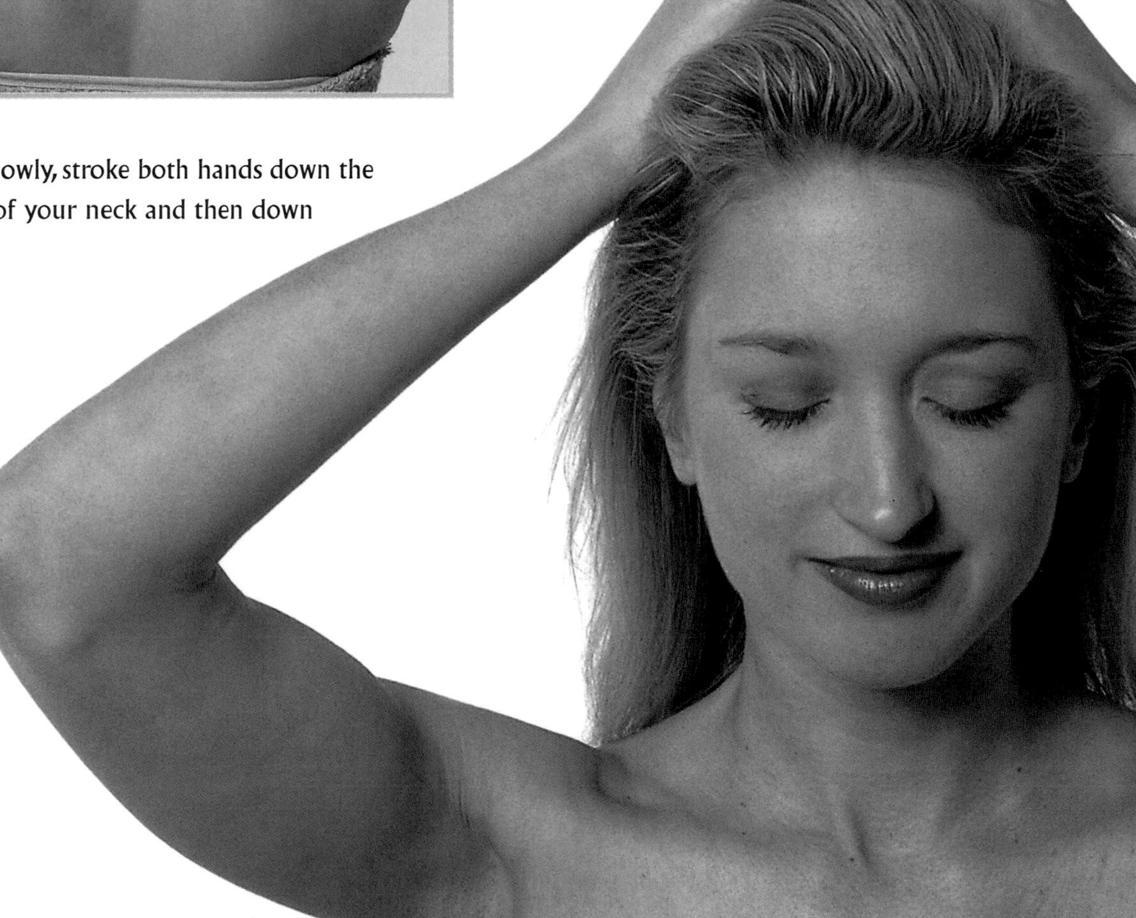

2 APPLYING FINGER-PAD FRICTION ('SHAMPOOING') TO YOUR SCALP

Place the pads of the fingers of both of your hands on top of your head and make small, circular movements over your entire scalp.

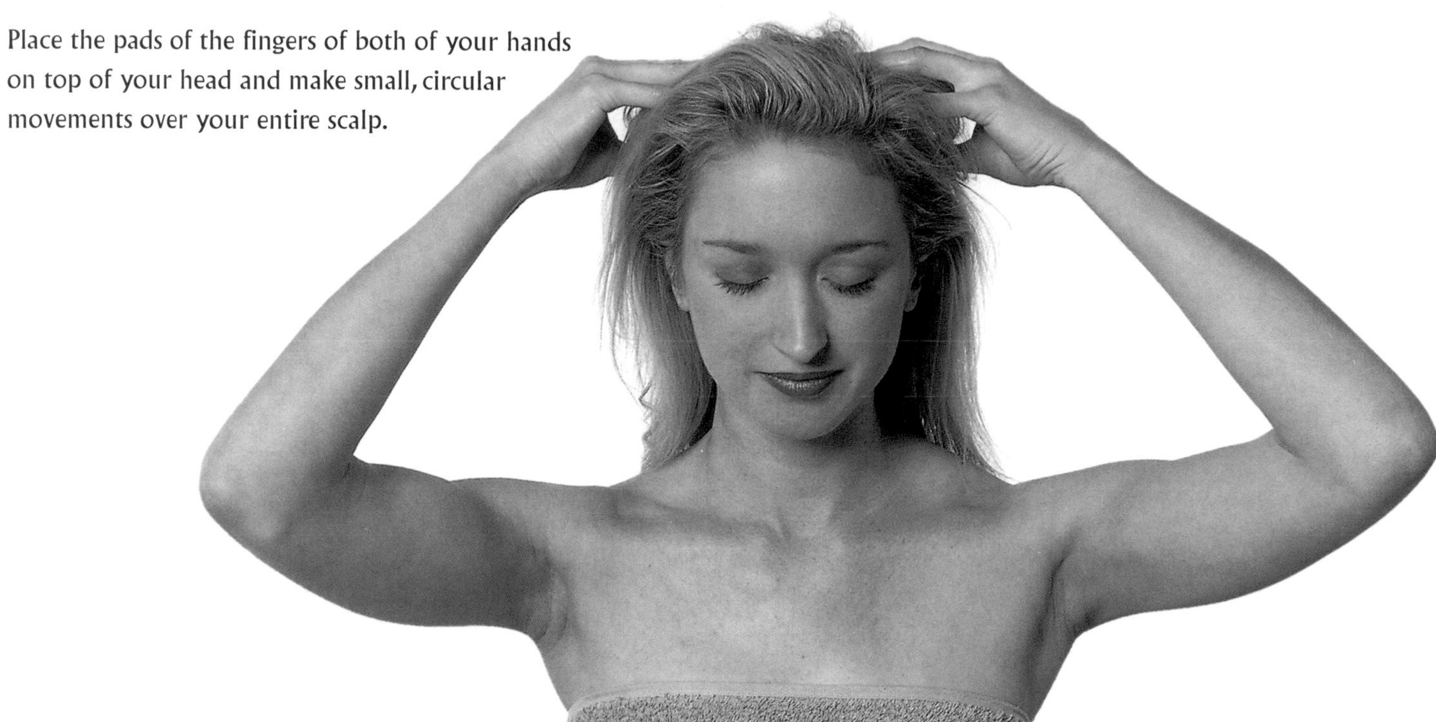

3 RUBBING YOUR SCALP

Place the palms of both of your hands on the crown of your head, with your fingers a few centimetres apart.

Perform brisk, light, rubbing movements over the top of your head. Continue by rubbing down the sides of your head.

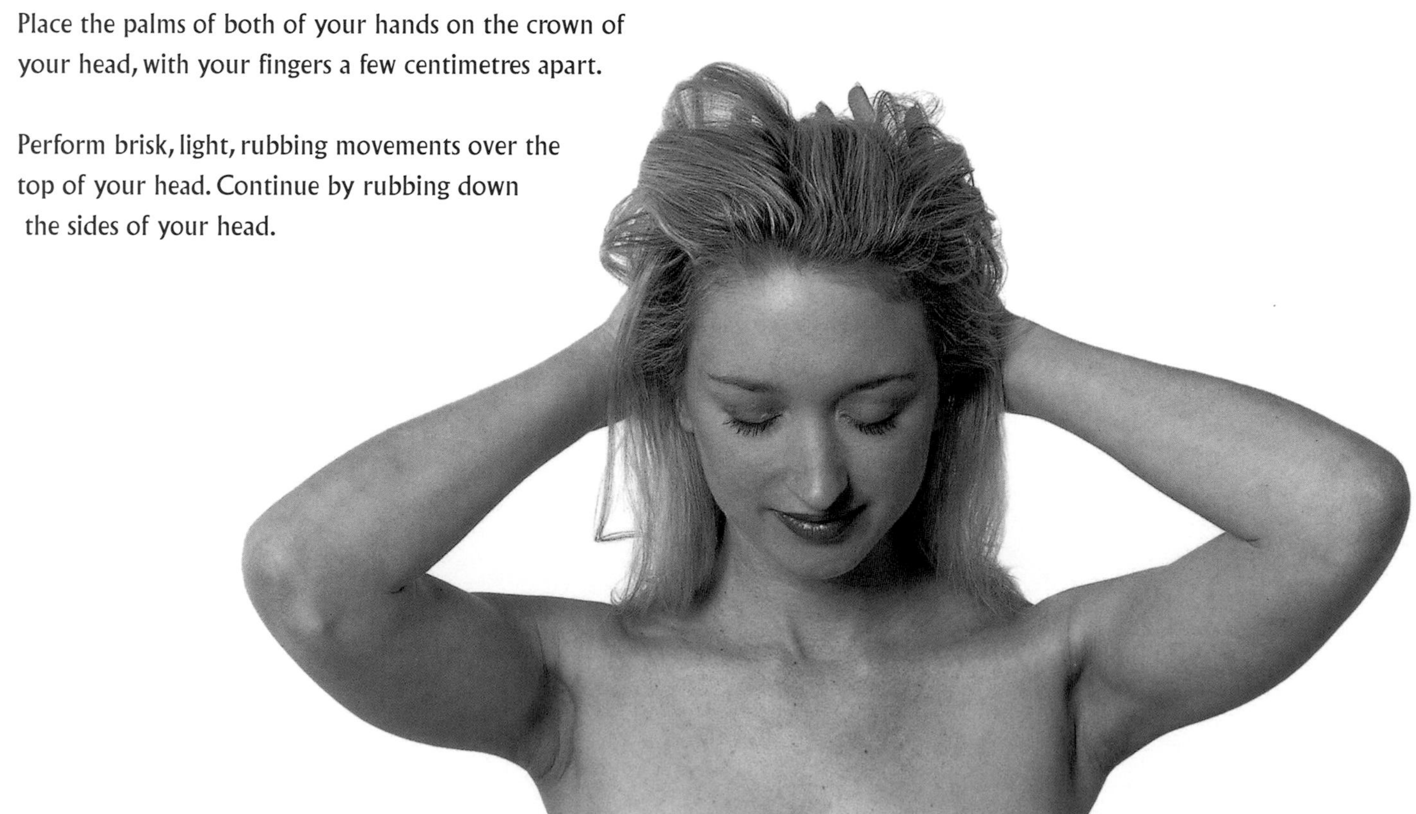

4 'COMBING' AND TUGGING YOUR HAIR

Using both of your hands, gently 'comb' your hair with your fingertips. Next try 'combing' your hair using one hand, followed by the other.

Form your hands into loose claw shapes, with your fingers spread out, and then gently place your fingers on your head. Gathering up small amounts of hair between your fingers and thumbs, gently tug your hair.

5 PLAYING ON YOUR SCALP

Use the pads of either only two fingers or all of them to tap (drum) over your entire head, bouncing off it lightly and rhythmically.

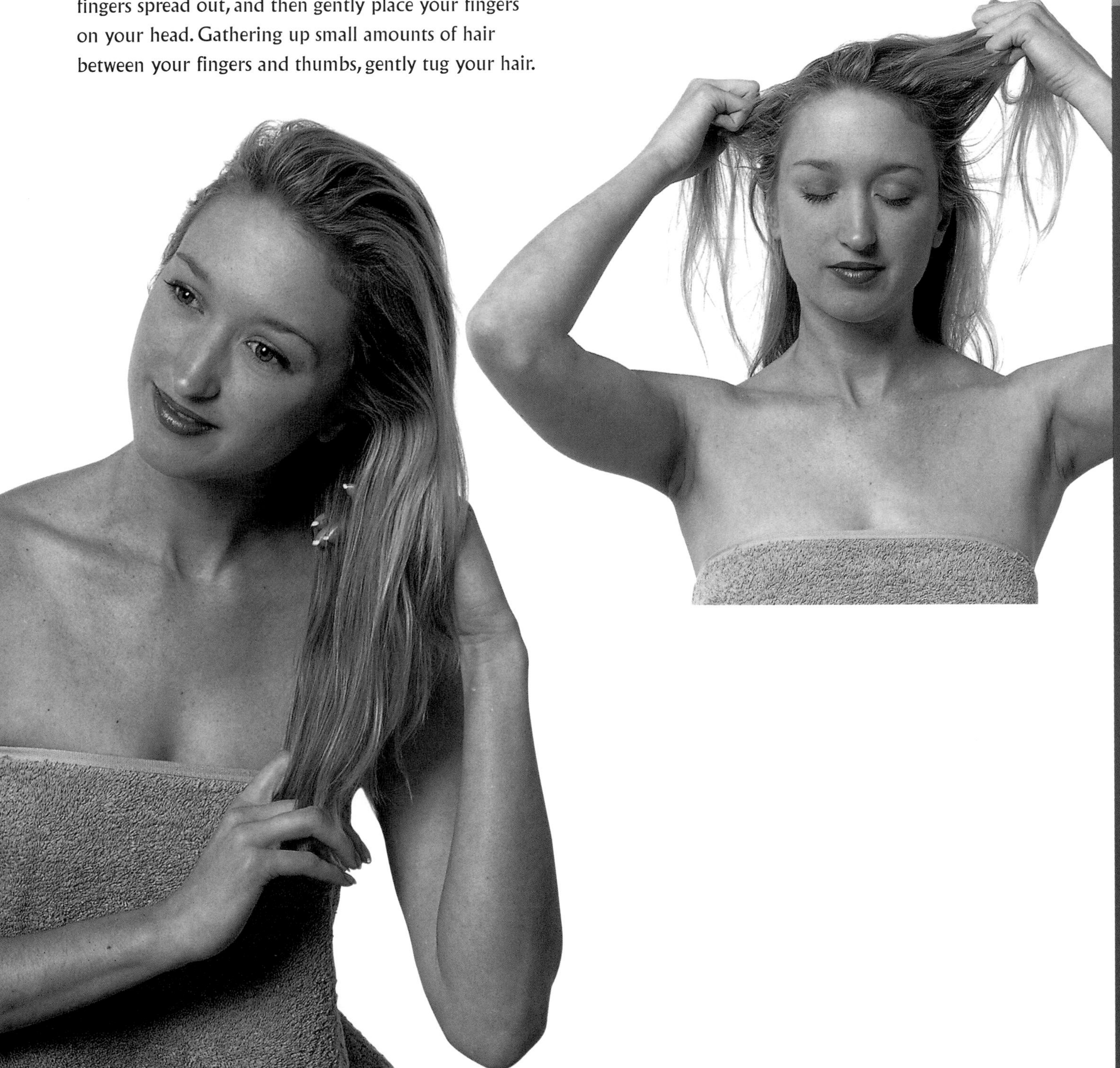

6 MASSAGING YOUR EARS

Place your index fingers on the front of each of your earlobes and your thumbs on the back. Working on both ears simultaneously, slowly massage all around them.

As you reach the top of your ears, tug them gently away from your head. Now lower your index fingers and thumbs to the middle of your ears and gently pull, and then tug, your earlobes.

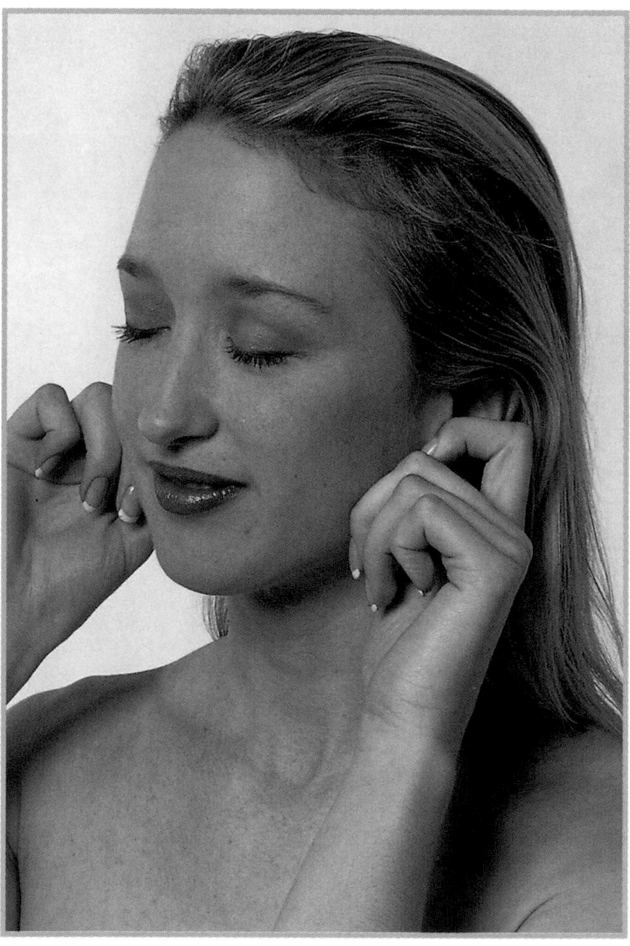

7 STROKING YOUR FACE

Place your hands on your forehead, with your fingertips pointing towards each other.

i) Stroke from the centre of your forehead outwards.

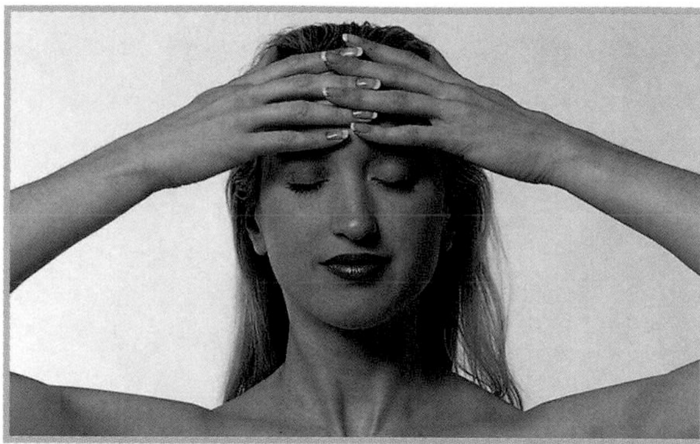

ii) Move your hands down to your cheeks. Now stroke from the sides of your nose outwards, towards your ears.

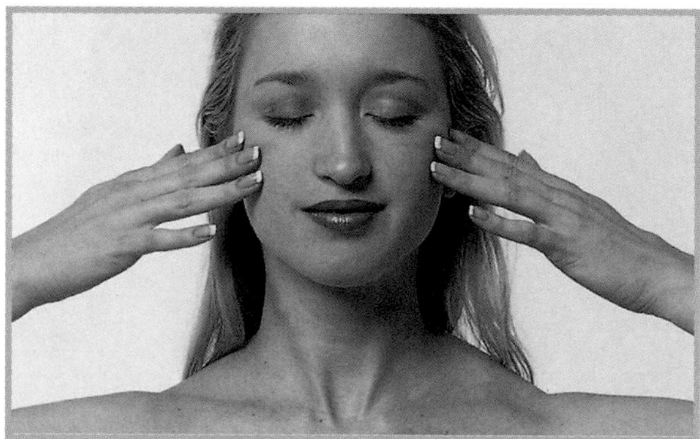

iii) Finally, move your hands down to your chin and again stroke outwards.

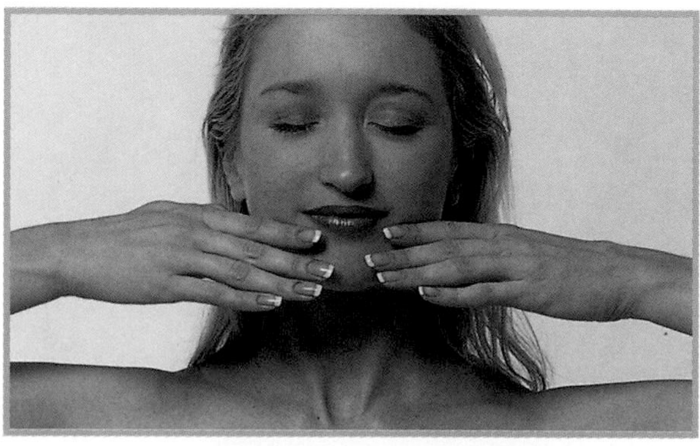

Repeat the above three procedures several times.

8 CIRCLING YOUR FACE

Position the fingertips of both hands in the centre of your forehead, just below the hairline.

Perform gentle, circular friction as you work down your forehead, cheeks and chin until you reach your jaw line.

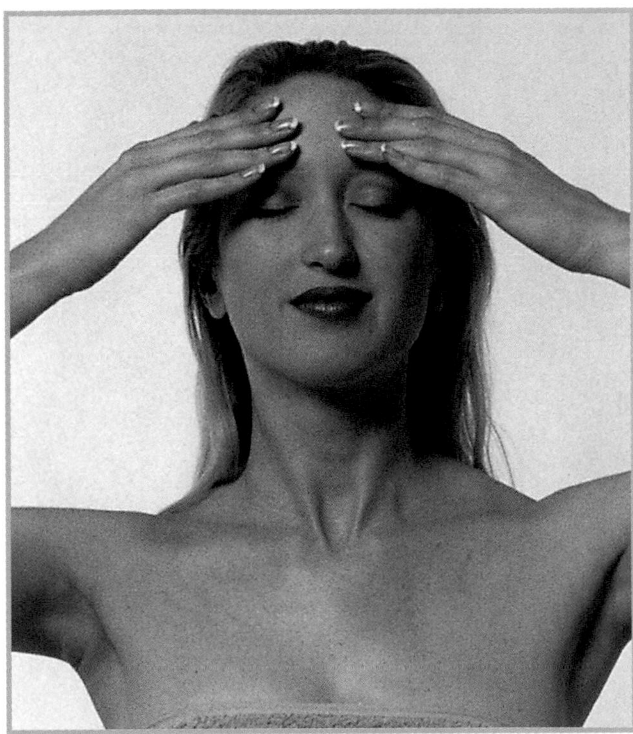

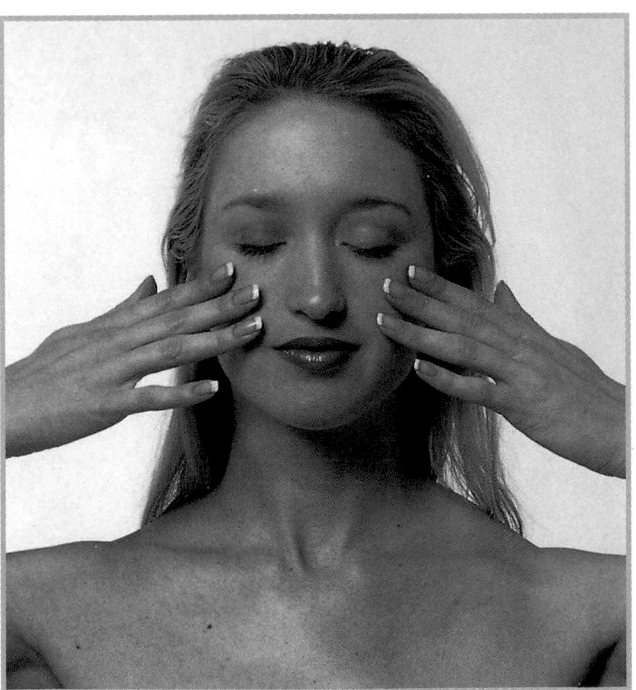

9 SQUEEZING YOUR EYEBROWS

Starting at the inner side of each eyebrow, gently squeeze all along your brow line using your thumbs and index fingers.

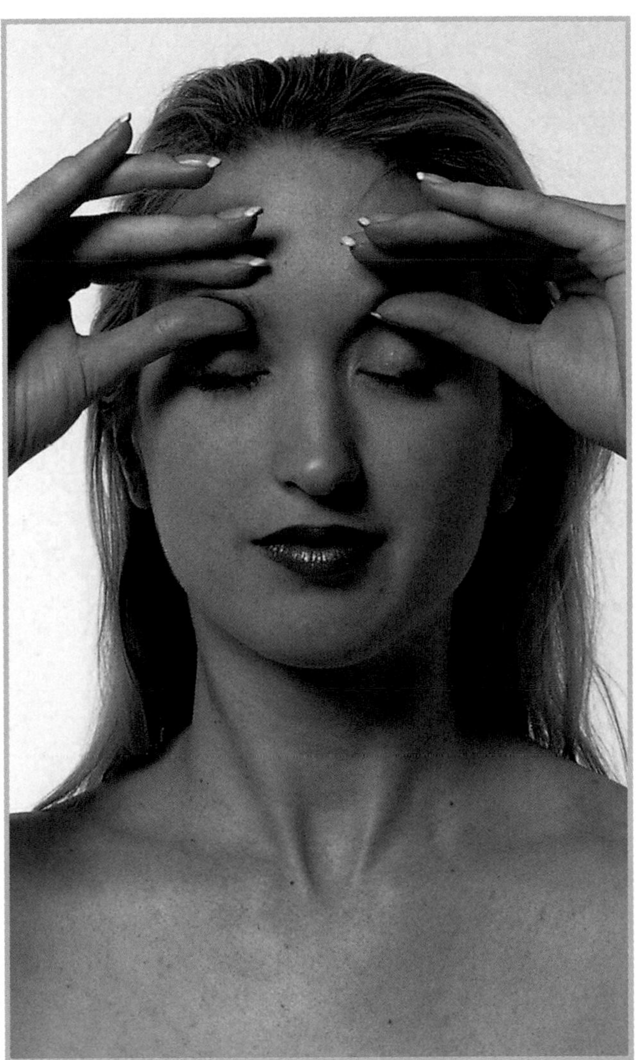

10 RELEASING JAW TENSION

Gently cup the centre of your jawbone between your thumbs and index fingers.

Then squeeze and release it. Working outwards along your jawbone, gently squeeze and release it at intervals of about two centimetres until you reach your ears.

11 CIRCLING YOUR EYES

Use the pads of your index and middle fingers to perform small, circular movements around both of your eyes.

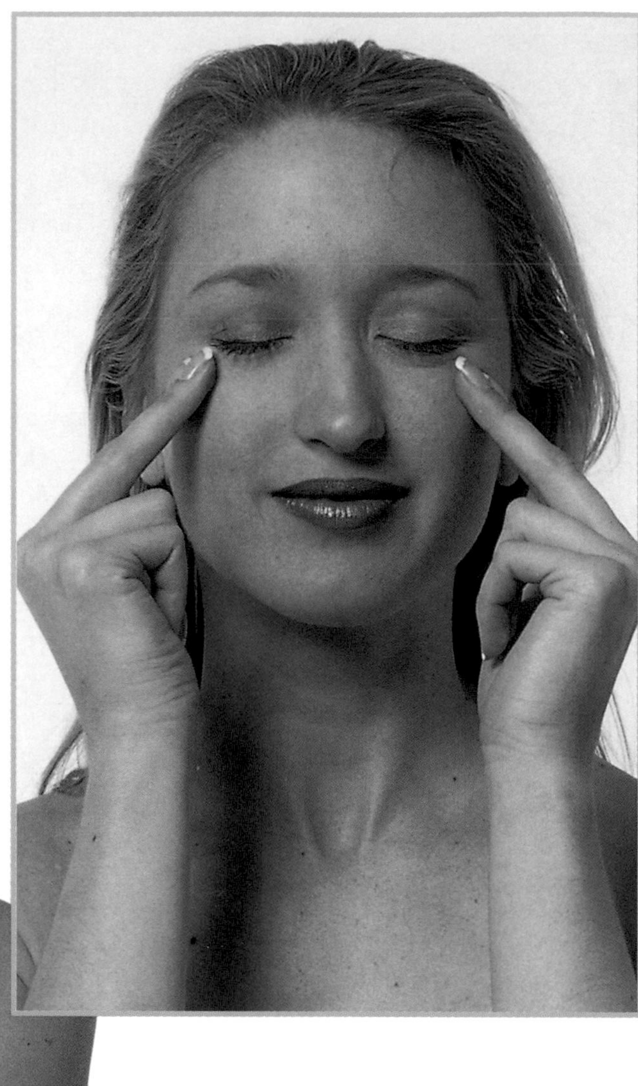

12 TAPPING YOUR FACE

Gently tap over all of your face using three or four fingertips. As you are doing this, keep your wrists loose and allow the pads of your fingers to bounce lightly off your skin.

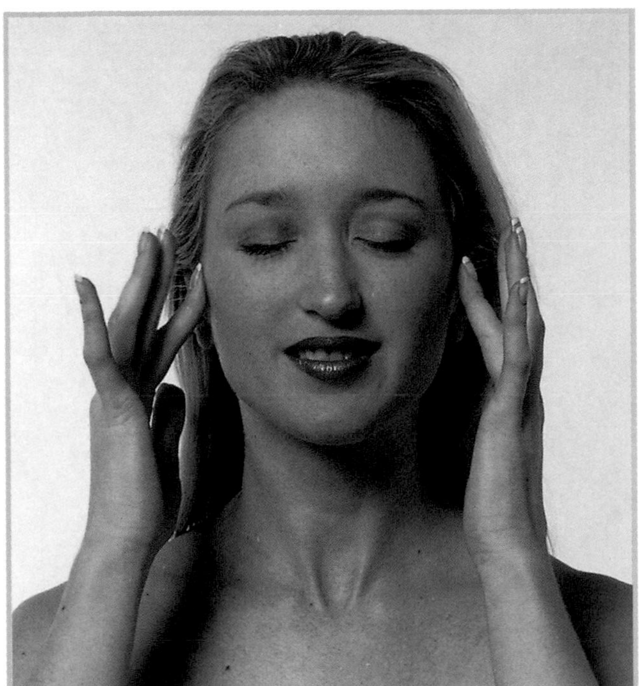

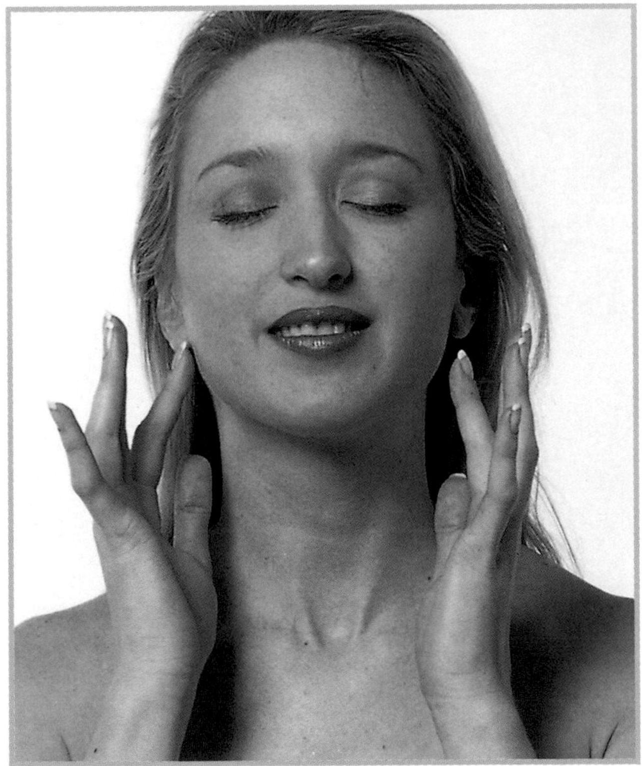

13 THE FINAL TOUCH

If your eyes are not already shut, close them gently.

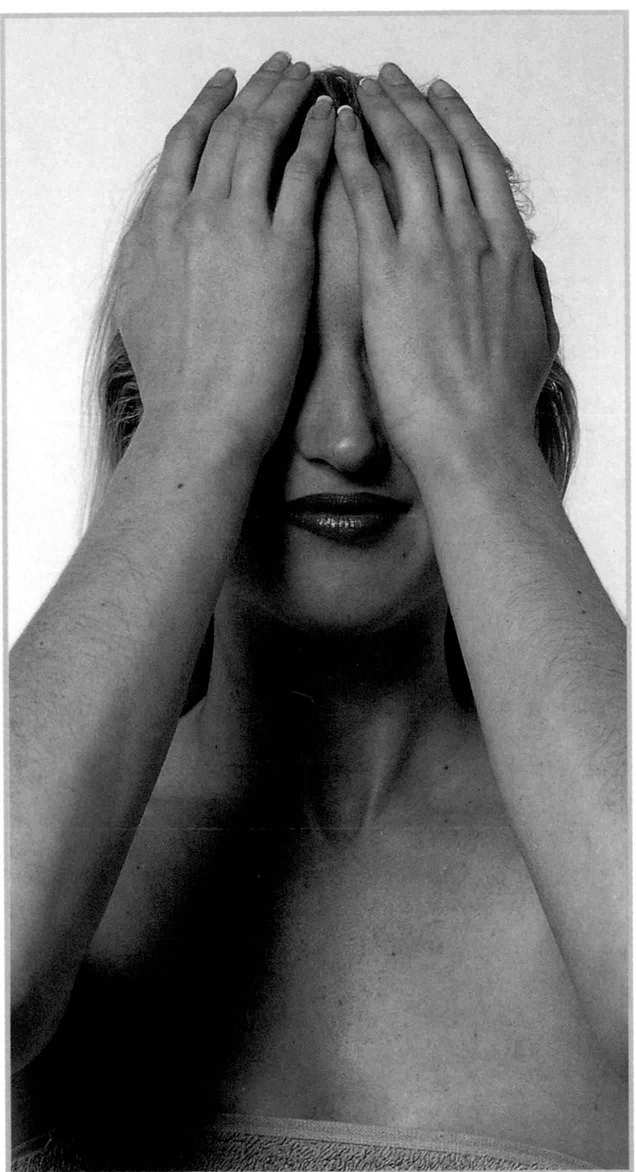

Gently place the palms of your hands, with your fingers pointing upwards, over your eyes. Feel how the heat and energy is relaxing and dissolving the tension in your eyes. Leave your hands over your eyes for as long as you like. When you finally take your hands away from your eyes, you should be feeling remarkably refreshed, yet also relaxed. Remember to drink lots of water and to follow the other aftercare instructions given on page 95. These, combined with regular Indian head massages, will help you to maintain excellent health.

Conclusion

I HOPE THAT YOU HAVE ENJOYED practising Indian head massage, on yourself and on your family and friends. If you practise it on a regular basis, you will experience an enormous difference in your health and well-being, not only physically, but emotionally.

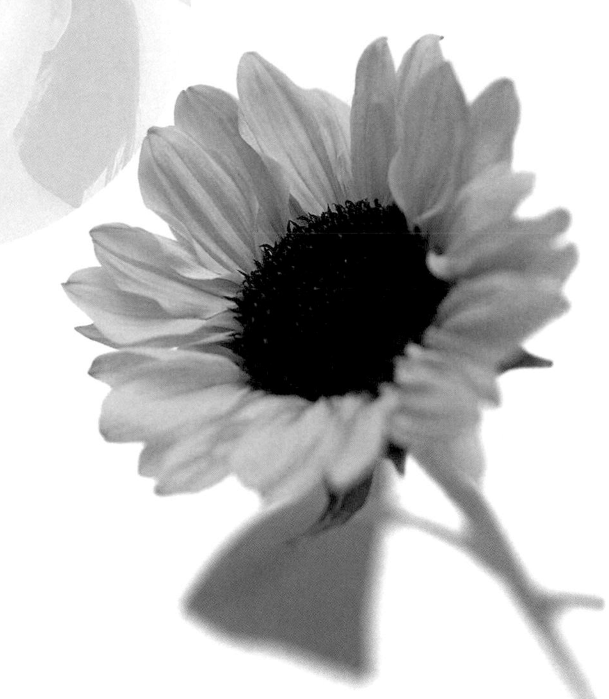

You may even wish to train to be a professional therapist. If so, there are many workshops that specialise in Indian head massage. Note, however, that a weekend course will not give you the necessary skills to become a qualified practitioner. A recognised professional course in Indian head massage should include a thorough initial grounding in anatomy and physiology. Once you are familiar with the structures and functions of the body, you will undertake practical tuition. You will also be expected to carry out case studies at home and to take exams in the theory and practice of Indian head massage.

Before signing up to it, ensure that a course is accredited to a professional association and that you are able to obtain insurance upon qualification. Study the

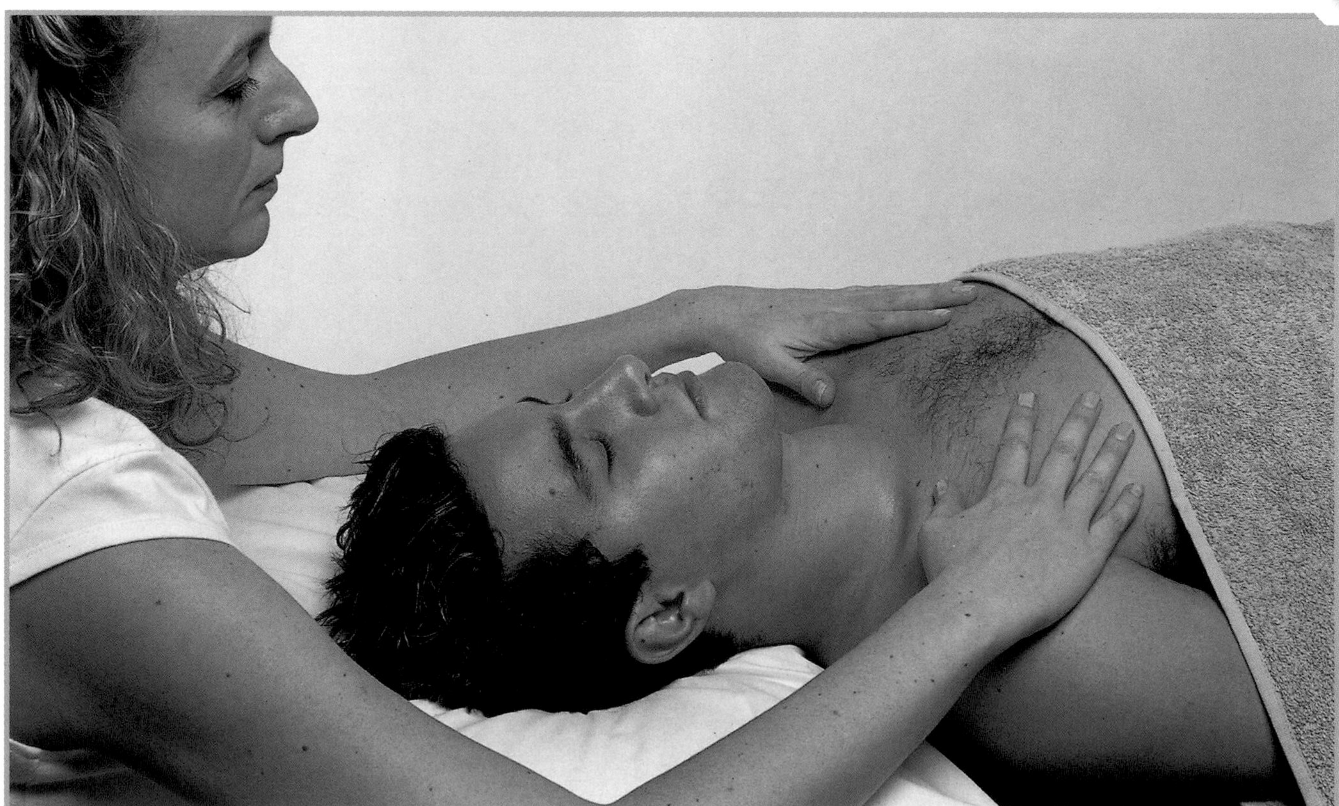

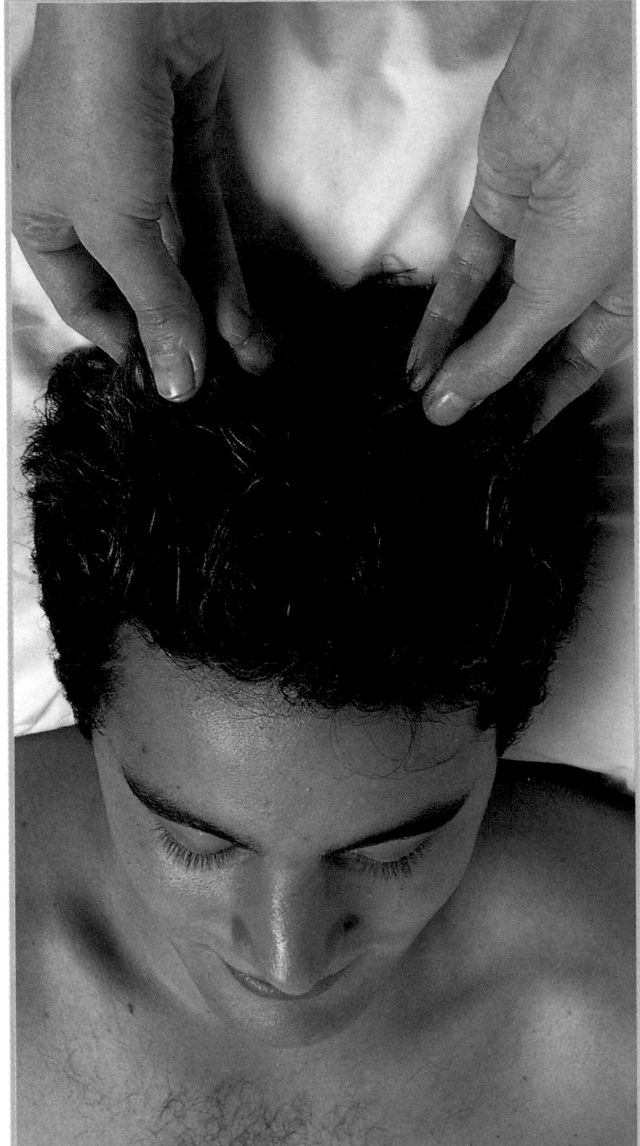

prospectuses of many colleges and do not be afraid to ask questions before making a commitment and parting with your money. How long has the college been established? What are the principal's qualifications and experience? How long has he or she been teaching? Is he or she still practising? Arrange to visit the college and to sit in on a lesson. Talk to the present students to find out if they are satisfied with the quality of the course and ask for recommendations.

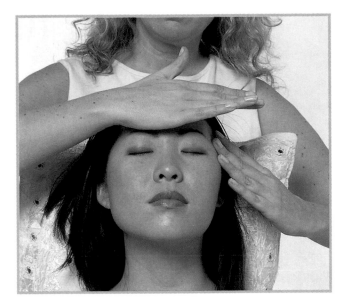

Complementary-health practitioners often combine Indian head massage with other therapies, such as massage, aromatherapy or reflexology. Indian head massage is an increasingly popular therapy, and qualified professionals work from home, in clinics, hospitals, health clubs, hospices, beauty salons, hairdressers', rehabilitation centres, airports, on cruise liners and so on. And, because Indian head massage may be performed anywhere, without requiring the receiver to disrobe, and takes just a short time to complete, therapists often visit offices.

Whether you practise this ancient healing art on yourself, your family and friends or practise it professionally, you will enjoy its rewards!

Index

Useful addresses

Beaumont College of Natural Medicine
MWB Business Exchange,
Hinton Road, Bournemouth BH1 2EF
Tel: +44 (0)1202 708887
Fax: +44 (0)1202 708720
http://www.beaumontcollege.co.uk
Information on training courses under the direction of Denise Brown.

Denise Brown Essential Oils
MWB Business Exchange,
Hinton Road, Bournemouth BH1 2EF
Tel: +44 (0)1202 708887
Fax: +44 (0)1202 708720
http://www.denisebrown.co.uk
A wide selection of high-quality, pure and unadulterated essential oils, base oils, creams, lotions and relaxation music is available from Denise Brown Essential Oils (international mail order).

Credits and acknowledgements

My thanks to David and Sarah of D&S Books for allowing me to write yet another book. My love and thanks to my dear husband, Garry, and to my two beloved children, Chloe and Thomas. Thanks also to all of my patients and students, who have taught me so much over the years.

Finally, I thank all of the higher energies of the cosmos that guide me in my work, especially Sai Baba and my angels and archangels. I feel truly blessed to be graced by their presence and unconditional love so that I may radiate fully the love and light of my being.

Picture credits

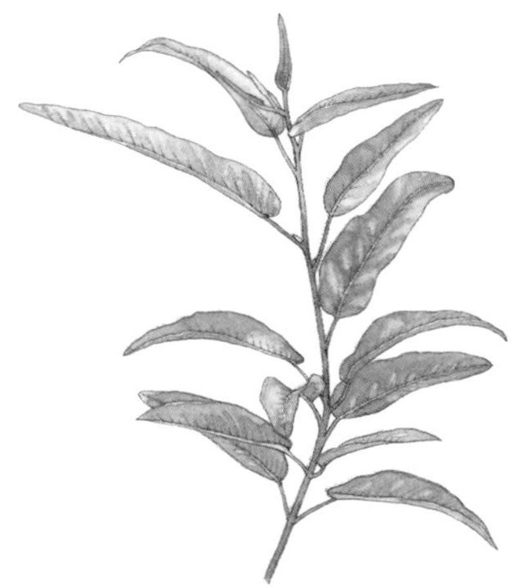